Ataxia - Practice Essentials and Interventions

Edited by Patricia Bozzetto Ambrosi

Published in London, United Kingdom

Ataxia - Practice Essentials and Interventions
http://dx.doi.org/10.5772/intechopen.104147
Edited by Patricia Bozzetto Ambrosi

Contributors
Bilal El-Mansoury, Jawad Laadraoui, Abdelaati El Khiat, Omar El Hiba, Arumugam R. Jayakumar, Abdessalam Ferssiwi, Abdelali Bitar, Barbara Pietrucha, Katerina Asonitou, Dimitra Koutsouki, Donnette A. Alicia Wright, Daniela Munoz Chesta, Monica Troncoso-Schifferli, Patricia Bozzetto Ambrosi, Caroline Bozzetto Ambrosi

First published in London, United Kingdom, 2024 by IntechOpen
IntechOpen is the global imprint of INTECHOPEN LIMITED, registered in England and Wales, registration number: 11086078, 5 Princes Gate Court, London, SW7 2QJ, United Kingdom

British Library Cataloguing-in-Publication Data
A catalogue record for this book is available from the British Library

Additional hard and PDF copies can be obtained from orders@intechopen.com

Ataxia - Practice Essentials and Interventions
Edited by Patricia Bozzetto Ambrosi
p. cm.
Print ISBN 978-1-83768-937-8
Online ISBN 978-1-83768-938-5
eBook (PDF) ISBN 978-1-83768-939-2

For EU product safety concerns:
IN TECH d.o.o., Prolaz Marije Krucifikse Kozulić 3, 51000 Rijeka, Croatia,
info@intechopen.com or visit our website at intechopen.com.

Meet the editor

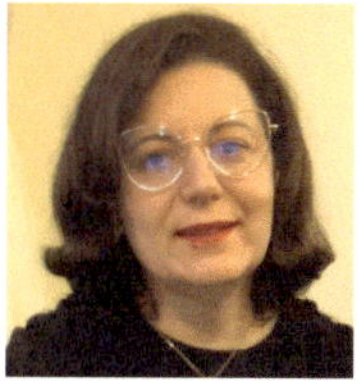

Prof. Dr. Patricia Bozzetto Ambrosi graduated in Medicine from the University of Caxias do Sul, Brazil, and the University of Rome Tor Vergata, Italy. She is a former researcher in Morphophysiology at the University of Córdoba/Reina Sofia Hospital, Córdoba, Spain. She obtained degrees in Neurology/Neurosurgery at the Hospital of Restauração, SES, Brazil, and Neuroradiology/Radiodiagnostics at Paris Marie Curie University (Sorbonne University), France. She holds a Master's Degree in Medicine from the University of Nova Lisboa, Portugal, and a Master's Degree in Behavioral Sciences and Neuropsychiatry from the University of Pernambuco, Brazil. She also has a Ph.D. in Biological Sciences from the University of Pernambuco/Paris Diderot University. She is a former fellow in Interventional Neuroradiology at the Ophthalmological Foundation Adolphe de Rothschild, Beaujon Hospital, and Hospices Civils de Strasbourg, France. She was Praticien Associé in Interventional Neuroradiology at Neurologique Hospital Pierre Wertheimer, University of Lyon Claude Bernard, France, and a visiting professor at the University of Paris Diderot-Neuri Beaujon, France. She is an independent Consultant in Neuroradiology, Endovascular Neurology, and Imaging, and a Clinical Professor of Medicine. She has also been an Academic Collaborator Researcher in the Cardiovascular Department at University of Leicester, England, and a Research Tutor at Sorbonne University, France. She has experience in innovative research for the development of new technologies and neurosciences and is an academic editor and reviewer of several scientific publications about neurological diseases.

Contents

Preface **IX**

Section 1
Introduction **1**

Chapter 1 **3**
Introductory Chapter: Insights into Ataxia
by Caroline Bozzetto Ambrosi and Patricia Bozzetto Ambrosi

Section 2
Common Scenarios **15**

Chapter 2 **17**
Ataxia Telangiectasia
by Barbara Pietrucha

Chapter 3 **41**
Childhood-Onset Ataxia
by Daniela Munoz Chesta and Mónica Troncoso-Schifferli

Chapter 4 **63**
Ataxia in Multiple Sclerosis: From Current Understanding to Therapy
by Bilal El-Mansoury, Jawad Laadraoui, Abdelaati El Khiat, Omar El Hiba, Arumugam R. Jayakumar, Abdessalam Ferssiwi and Abdelali Bitar

Section 3
Interventions **89**

Chapter 5 **91**
Adapted Physical Activity and Ataxia
by Katerina Asonitou and Dimitra Koutsouki

Chapter 6 **111**
Nutritional Care and Intervention in Spinocerebellar Ataxia
by Donnette A. Wright

Preface

Ataxia or dystaxia is a disorder of the nervous system characterized by a lack of coordination of voluntary muscle movements and imbalance. It is normally associated with degeneration or blockage of specific areas of the cerebrum, cerebellum, and/or vestibular sensory connection pathways with the periphery.

Among all neurological diseases, ataxia stands out for its considerable variability of causes. There may be numerous etiologies for ataxias, and they may occur alone or simultaneously, acutely or chronically, and at any age in children, adults, and the elderly. As the pathophysiology of ataxias is as diverse as the various neurological and systemic diseases that affect the nervous system, the first step is to discover its underlying mechanism and rule out a detectable known genetic cause. Non-genetic ataxias are caused by acquired conditions, sporadic neurodegenerative disorders, or by unknown processes.

This book unravels the foundations and essential interventions of ataxia disorders, presenting introductory and pathophysiological aspects to give an overview of ataxia as well as contemporary and current evidence-based information on various scenarios, for example, when the disorder appears during early childhood, or even in adulthood and old age, in addition to presenting the authors' views and guidelines for interventions based on their own experiences.

The first section consists of an introductory chapter that gives an overview of ataxic disease that mainly affects adults. It discusses the main processes that cause ataxia, the most common signs and symptoms, what is involved in the ataxic patient, ataxia's variability, the main diagnostic tests used, and the treatment of ataxia in adults.

The second section focuses on several common scenarios in which the ataxic disorder will appear. Chapter 2 discusses genetic conditions like ataxia telangiectasia, which is an autosomal recessive disorder characterized by cerebellar degeneration, telangiectasias, immunodeficiency, cancer susceptibility, and radiation sensitivity. Ataxia telangiectasia is a complex disorder that usually first appears in early childhood when children begin to sit or walk. Although the disease is genetic, there are still many unresolved questions about its complexity and severity, for example, the influence of environmental factors, disease-modifying genes, epigenetics, severity, and progression of its various manifestations. Chapter 3 gives an overview of childhood-onset ataxia disorder. Childhood presentations of ataxia can often be difficult to diagnose. Recognizing ataxia is especially difficult in young children; the most frequent reason for consultation is gait instability and loss of balance. Clinical presentations tend to be heterogeneous and key considerations may vary based on age of onset, disease progression, and associated manifestations. New genetic diagnosis techniques have emerged, enabling the identification of specific pathologies. While there are currently limited treatable conditions, ongoing studies are proposing promising treatments for certain pathologies in the near future, thus increasing the importance of accurate diagnostic approaches. Chapter 4 is about neurodegenerative diseases, such as multiple sclerosis, in which ataxia is a common neurological manifestation affecting about 80% of people with the disease, in addition to being a symptom that can drastically affect the patient's quality of life. The underlying pathophysiology of ataxia in multiple sclerosis is not fully understood, but it is thought to be related to demyelination and neurodegeneration in specific areas of the brain. These symptoms can range from mild to severe and can include lack of coordination, difficulty speaking and difficulty walking. Therapeutic interventions usually involve pharmacotherapy to improve coordination, physical therapy to increase strength and balance, surgical procedures to relieve tremors, and occupational therapy. It is important to work closely with a clinician to develop a personalized plan to treat symptoms.

The last section deals with interventions and therapies and includes two chapters detailing various therapies for ataxia to improve quality of life. Chapter 5 examines physical therapy and nutritional therapy, and Chapter 6 reviews common treatment options used concurrently with drug therapy to control symptoms.

There are currently no specific approved therapies for the treatment of ataxia, however, several promising therapeutic approaches are being investigated, including the use of disease-modifying therapies, rehabilitation interventions, and symptomatic treatments. Many research efforts are underway to find more effective treatments for ataxia, including rehabilitation measures that can be done at home to help maintain the patient's muscle strength and balance.

Dr. Patricia Bozzetto Ambrosi
Independent Clinical Neurology and Imaging Consultant,
London, United Kingdom

Clinical Professor,
European Academy of Neurology,
London, United Kingdom

Academic Researcher Fellow,
International Association of Hospice and Palliative Care,
London, United Kingdom

Member of National Ataxia Foundation,
London, United Kingdom

Section 1

Introduction

Chapter 1

Introductory Chapter: Insights into Ataxia

Caroline Bozzetto Ambrosi and Patricia Bozzetto Ambrosi

1. Introduction

The term "ataxia" or also "distaxia" means the inability to coordinate, but at the same time, it is also used to describe the group of underlying neurological disorders that affect coordination, balance, and speech. The delineation of ataxic disorders as distinct entities can be said to have begun with the description of siblings with ataxia by Nicholas Friedreich in the 1860s, suggesting a genetic etiology, though there are possible descriptions of similar disorders antedating this [1–3].

Ataxic disorders also refer to symptoms that affect the coordination of these movements. They may be a symptom of several degenerative medical or neurological conditions of the nervous system that compromise the movements of different regions of the body — fingers, hands, arms, legs, eyes, balance, muscle tone, swallowing, and speech. It can also be manifested as a lack of coordination that impairs voluntary movement as a whole. The common symptoms of ataxia are similar to those of a drunk such as slurred speech, stumbling, falling, and incoordination [4, 5].

The number of ataxia subtypes is unknown, but it is estimated that there are at least 100 different subtypes, each with a distinct etiology. To date, current classifications subdivide ataxias into three large groups: (i) degenerative ataxias, (ii) hereditary ataxias, and (iii) acquired ataxias related to exogenous or endogenous non-genetic insults [5].

The purpose of this chapter is to provide a brief introduction for academics and clinicians with introductory tips for understanding, evaluating, and managing ataxias in general.

2. Pathophysiology of ataxia

Ataxic disease is most commonly caused by dysfunction of the cerebellum or its pathways, including impairment of vestibular or proprioceptive input to the cerebellum [6, 7]. Cerebro-cerebellar connectivity is organized into multiple circuits that function to connect devices in parallel. Depending on the location of the cerebro-cerebellar connectivity injury, the characteristic findings regarding ataxic disorders are generally the following: Lesions affecting the lateral portion of the cerebellum lead to ipsilateral symptoms, while lesions affecting diffusely can lead to generalized symptoms. Lesions affecting the cerebellar hemisphere lead to appendicular ataxia. While insults within the vermis lead to postural gait ataxia with limb preservation. Lesions in the vestibulocerebellar areas cause gait imbalance, vertigo, and ataxia [8–10].

IntechOpen

Taking into account the clinical scenario, according to Cabaraux et al., 2021, cerebellar symptoms of cerebellar injury can be grouped into three main cerebellar syndromes:

1. Cerebellar Motor Syndrome, when lesions generally affect the lobes I-V, VI, and VIII and where patients present different combinations of speech alterations (scanned, explosive, and nasal voice), mutism, limb ataxia with loss of coordination (dysmetria, dysdiadochokinesia, tremor, hypotonia, cerebellar convulsions, and other related conditions), defective writing, gait staggering, and steadiness and impaired motor skills.

2. Vestibulocerebellar Syndrome when injuries occur in the vestibular nuclei that are connected to lobes IX–X and the dorsal oculomotor vermis corresponding to lobes V–VII are affected in these cases and is characterized by various combinations of dysmetria, saccadic pursuit, nystagmus, impaired vestibulo-ocular vision, oblique gaze deviation [8, 11, 12].

3. Schmahmann Syndrome or Cerebellar Cognitive-Affective Syndrome when lesions affect lobes VI-IX and patients present different combinations of dysexecutive, visuospatial, linguistic deficits and affective dysregulation that is characterized by changes in executive functions (management, factual situation, abstraction, verbal fluency, memory) and may also present a lack of attention; disorganization and affected visuospatial memory; personality change with affective changes and inappropriate behavior; and language difficulties [13–15].

The ataxic diseases can generally be the result of a considerable variability of causes, and there can be numerous etiologies for ataxias, which can occur isolated or simultaneously, acutely or chronically, and at any age, both in children and in adults and even common in the elderly [6–10].

Findings from the physical examination, in combination with the assessment of risk factors and presentation of the complaint, lead to a decision. Ataxia also can be seen in 30–60% of patients with posterior circulation stroke [14, 15]. Patients may present atypically and with multiple causes that may exist simultaneously. This contributes to the important clinical heterogeneity of ataxic disorders in daily practice [8].

However, studies have shown that misdiagnoses of posterior circulation strokes are frequent, with dizziness and difficulty walking more likely to be manifested than focal weakness, changes in vision, or neglect [10–15]. In emergency care, attention should be focused on treatable and reversible etiologies of ataxia.

Hereditary ataxias represent a wide clinical spectrum of disorders, and phenotypic variability is recurrent between individuals suffering from the same ataxia subtype. It may be characterized by episodic, spinocerebellar, Friedreich's, X-linked, and mitochondrial ataxia as well as sporadic conditions. Clinically, it is presented by progressive ataxia combined with extra-cerebellar and multisystemic involvements, including peripheral neuropathy, pyramidal signs, movement disorders, seizures, and cognitive dysfunction. Friedreich's ataxia is the most common cause of an autosomal recessive pattern of inheritance, appearing between the first and second decades of life. The abnormalities affecting multisystem are seen and include myocardiopathy, endocrinological diseases, vision, and hearing loss. Gait ataxia, loss of sensory and proprioception, *pes cavus*, spastic extensor plantar responses, and extremities atrophies [6, 16, 17].

3. Common signs and symptoms and clinical assessment

On the physical examination of neurological ataxic patients, one of the main neurological symptoms and signs to be investigated when locating lesions in the nervous system with a complete neurological examination. Recognizing its importance becomes crucial, especially when it comes to changes in gait, changes in speech, and abnormal eye movements. Another ability to research related to ataxia refers to the inability to coordinate the position of the head, trunk, and limbs. Ataxia can also be a sensory dysfunction, and not just a motor one, which can only be identified when the patient moves. Remember that it can also be confused with motor impairment [18]. However, the main difference between ataxia and paresis is that ataxia affects coordination without affecting strength, while paresis affects only strength, and they are often confused with each other. However, the type of ataxia is characterized by a complete neurological examination (mental status, gait – postural reactions (mainly), assessment of cranial nerves, spinal reflexes, and pain perception), and the main causes of ataxia can be separated into vestibular, sensory ataxia, cerebellar, and antalgic [19].

Common signs and symptoms of ataxic patients include gait abnormalities, slurred speech, difficulty walking, abnormal eye movements, difficulty swallowing, increased fatigue, incoordination in fine motor movements such as handwriting, buttoning shirts, typing, tremors, vertigo, and cognition problems [20]. Clinicians should ask patients whether any of the signs and symptoms are present, the level of functional disability in activities of daily living, onset, and progression. At this point, the clinical assessment of ataxia can be performed by a set of ataxia rating scales [21].

There are several ataxia rating scales based on different ataxic populations, and four scales are highlighted following:

1. Scale for Assessment and Rating of Ataxia – SARA [22]

2. International Cooperative Ataxia Rating Scales – ICARS [23]

3. Friedreich's Ataxia Rating Scale – FARS [24]

4. Unified Multiple System Atrophy Rating Scale – UMSARS [25]

Ataxia evaluative scales have psychometric properties such as feasibility, acceptability, consistency, and reproducibility. They are usually used in different ataxic populations [21] in a way that determines similarities and differences in the aspects of ataxia addressed. For example, SARA mainly assesses ataxia and motor performance, while ICARS is concerned with assessing vision and ocular motricity disorders. Autonomic functions and bulbar dysfunctions are assessed in both UMSARS and FARS. The SARA scale proves to be an ideal scale for rapid assessment of ataxia or in clinical settings that require rapid screening. UMSARS or FARS are more appropriate for assessing the impact of ataxia on general health, monitoring the progression of ataxia, activity of daily living, and the individual's disability [26].

4. Essential evaluation and differential diagnosis

The progression of ataxia from symptom onset to maximum deficit is to be known whether it is acquired, genetic or non-hereditary sporadic degenerative.

Acquired ataxias usually present acutely and progress rapidly from vascular, immune-mediated, infectious, and toxic causes. Substrate deficiencies (e.g., vitamin B1, B12, E, or A) and iatrogenic insults, other than acute drug overdose, present subacutely (**Table 1**) [27, 28].

A detailed history should be obtained to assist in identifying the cause of the ataxia. A detailed history and physical and neurological examinations should be performed. Neurological examination allows the clinician to identify the type of ataxia. Once the type of ataxia has been identified, other diagnostic tests should be performed according to the type of ataxia and the location of the lesion. Although most patients with ataxia have a primary neurological disease, it is important to know the cause can be metabolic disorders (e.g., hypoglycemia and hypocalcemia), toxins (e.g., lead and organophosphates), and medications (e.g., phenobarbital and metronidazole). Once a detailed history is obtained, physical and neurological examinations should be performed. The neurological examination can help clinicians to identify the type of ataxia. Once the type of ataxia is presumed, further diagnostic tests can be performed according to the type of ataxia and the lesion localization suspected [27].

Congenital diseases are also important causes of ataxia, specifically chronic ataxic syndromes such as Dandy–Walker Syndrome and Arnold Chiari Malformations. The Dandy–Walker syndrome is characterized by enlargement of the fourth ventricle in the posterior fossa, absence of the cerebellar vermis, and a cystic formation close to the internal base of the skull [28]. In Arnold Chiari malformations, the affected patient shows a downward displacement of the cerebellar tonsils through the foramen magnum with a presumed risk of complicating with a non-obstructive hydrocephalus [29].

Genetic ataxias can be highlighted as an autosomal dominant, autosomal recessive, or X-linked manner inheritance. The presence of a genetic disease does not exclude

Subtype	Etiology or related agent
Congenital	Developmental
Mass lesion	Tumor, Cyst, Aneurysm, Hematoma, Abscess, Normal Pressure, or Partial Obstructive Hydrocephalus
Vascular	Stroke, Hemorrhage, Subcortical Vascular Disease
Infections	Anthrax, Epstein–Barr, enterovirus, HIV, HTLV, Prion disease, Lyme Disease, Syphilis, Measles, Rubella, Varicella, Whipple's Disease, and Progressive Multifocal Leukoencephalopathy
External causes	Post-Anoxic, Post-Hyperthermic, Post-Traumatic
Epilepsy	Long-Standing Epilepsy
Systemic	Acute Thiamine (B1) Deficiency, Chronic Vitamin B12 and E Deficiencies, Autoimmune Thyroiditis, and Low Thyroids Levels
Toxic	Common Drug Reaction (Amiodarone, Cytosine Arabinoside, 5-Fluorouracil, Lithium, Phenytoin, Valproic acid} Environmental (Acrylamide, Alcohol, Organic Solvents, Organo-lead/Mercury/Tin, and Inorganic Bismuth/Mercury/Thallium)
Immunological	Vasculitis (Giant Cell Arteritis, Behcet's disease, Systemic Lupus Erythematosus, and others). Paraneoplastic (Anti-Yo, Hu, Ri, Ma Ta, CV2, Zic4, Anti-calcium channel, Anti-CRMP-5, ANNA-1,2,3; mGluR1, and TR). Autoimmune disorders (Anti-GluR2,GAD, MPP1, GD1b ganglioside, and anti-gliadin)

Adapted from Evaluation and Management of Ataxic Disorders [27, p. 2].

Table 1.
Identifiable causes for non-hereditary ataxia.

the presence of an acquired etiology that may alter the presentation and course of ataxia symptoms and warrant further investigation. Likewise, the absence of a clear family history does not exclude the role of genetics within an apparently sporadic disorder. Often, the fact that family history has not been adequately obtained because the information is not straight available (adoption, loss of contact, non-cooperation, and paternity issues), due to non-dominant inheritance patterns (recessive, X-linked, and maternal/mitochondrial) or due to specific genetic processes that modify the presentation of the disease in the pedigree (anticipation, incomplete penetrance, and mosaicism) [24].

Adult-onset genetic ataxias may not appear to clinicians until later in the course of the disease due to their insidious onset and slow progression.

Progressive muscular atrophy appears much more quickly compared to tardive idiopathic ataxia and genetic ataxia, causing significant disability in a short space of time, with death occurring 6–10 years after the onset of symptoms. Genetic counseling and risk assessment depend on determining the specific cause of hereditary ataxia in an individual.

5. Variability in rate or progression

The ataxia disorders may be associated with very specific causes. When the onset of symptoms occurs acutely and abruptly, it may be related to vascular and/or structural brain damage. While rapid onset over hours-days is more associated with infectious or parainfectious cerebellitis, immune-mediated diseases such as Miller–Fisher syndrome, acute exposure to toxins, metabolic insult, or multiple sclerosis [27, 28]. Onset that occurs over weeks to months is associated with paraneoplastic disorders: anti-glutamic acid decarboxylase antibody syndrome, steroid-responsive encephalopathy and ataxia, gluten ataxia in celiac disease, vitamin deficiency states, general medical conditions such as hepatic encephalopathy, infections, sensory polyneuropathy, and ganglionopathy.

The long-standing progression occurring over the years is associated with genetic ataxias and may vary according to the individual: toxins, multiple sclerosis, storage disorders, sporadic neurodegenerative disorders, atypical parkinsonian conditions such as progressive supranuclear palsy or neurosyphilis. All possible etiologies must be considered when the clinical course is not fully determined. They must be differentiated from disorders such as dystonia, parkinsonism, chorea, myoclonus, cognitive impairment, pyramidal signs, sensory loss, hyporeflexia, cognitive and psychiatric symptoms, eye movement abnormalities, visual loss, neuromuscular deficits, telangiectasias, Achilles xanthomas, and early cataracts [30].

6. Further diagnostic tests

The following diagnostic tests as magnetic resonance imaging of the brain and spine, in addition to serum tests that can be indicated and guided by clinical and imaging evaluation, studies of the cerebrospinal fluid are obtained for paraneoplastic, immune-mediated, infectious and inflammatory disorders: protein, glucose, different blood count, cultures, IgG synthesis, index, rate; oligoclonal bands, cytology, lactate, 14-3-3 protein, paraneoplastic antibodies; viral encephalitis panel and Venereal Disease Research Laboratory test levels.

• MRI brain and spinal cord, with and without contrast, with diffusion-weighted imaging (DWI) sequences
• Additional imaging:. MR spectroscopy or positron emission tomography (PET) scan/dopa-PET scan
• Electroencephalogram and Evoked Potentials (Visual, Auditory, Somatosensory)
• Electromyogram with nerve conduction studies
• Chest X-ray
• *First-line lab checks*: CBC, chemistry panel, HgbA1c, fasting lipids, ERS, ANA, RPR, TSH; vitamin E, folic acid, and vitamin B12 levels; methylmalonic acid, homocysteine, and urine heavy metals
• *Second-line lab checks*: CPK, SPEP, postprandial lactate-pyruvate-ammonia, ketones, copper, ceruloplasmin, zinc, ACE, Lyme diseases titers, HTLV I/II, HIV, anti-thyroid antibodies, anti-gliadin antibodies (and anti-endomysial/anti transglutaminase antibodies), anti-GAD antibodies (and anti amphiphysin antibodies)
• *Third line lab checks*: very long chain fatty acids/phytanic acid, urine and plasmatic amino acids, urine organic acids, lysosomal hydrolase screen including hexosaminidase A, coenzyme Q10 levels, glutathione levels, PRPN gene analysis
• *Spinal fluid studies*: cell count, glucose, lactate, protein, VDRL, gram stain, cultures as appropriate, cryptococcal antigen, 14-3-3 protein, neuron-specific enolase, prion protein studies, neurotransmitter levels as appropriate, myelin basic protein, oligoclonal bands, IgG synthesis
• *Biopsies*: conjunctival, muscle/nerve, GI tract, bone marrow, brain
• *Paraneoplastic workup*: tailored imaging(ultrasound, CT, and MRI), alpha fetoprotein, paraneoplastic antibodies (Yo, Hu, Ri, CV2, MaTa, Zic4, and others)
• *Genetic workup if no family history of ataxia*: Gene tests for SCA6, SCA3, SCA1, Friedreich ataxia, and fragile X-associated tremor/ataxia syndrome. Inborn errors of metabolism. Clinical whole exome sequencing
Adapted from Evaluation and Management of Ataxic Disorders [27, p. 4].

Table 2.
Workup for patients with ataxic disorders.

In case of suspicion of occult malignancy, a CT scan or PET scan of the body may be indicated. Further diagnostic testing that may be helpful in certain situations includes electroencephalogram, electromyography, nerve conduction studies, autonomic studies, or sleep studies. In selected cases, nerve, muscle, and brain biopsies are used for suspected mitochondrial ataxias in leukodystrophies or idiopathic etiology. Other rarely indicated tests include magnetic resonance spectroscopy imaging of the brain and dopamine transporter single photon emission computed tomography (SPECT) (DaT) scan (abnormal in MSA-C and other specific illnesses). Specialized genetic testing for inborn errors of metabolism, leukodystrophies, and storage disorders should be ordered if the remainder of the evaluation raises suspicions about these rare conditions. The patient should be adequately counseled about the implications and costs of genetic testing before ordering [6, 27]. Several sporadic ataxias do not have an identified cause. When followed over time, about one-third of Idiopathic Late Onset Cerebellar Ataxia can progress to MSA-C. Unidentified genetic mutations may be responsible for the remainder of ataxias (**Table 2**) [28, 31].

7. Treatment and management

Specific interventions include steroids for paraneoplastic and other immunological disorders as well as immunomodulatory therapies for steroid-responsive encephalopathy associated with Hashimoto's encephalopathy. General measures include eliminating toxins, compensating metabolic states, and treating deficiency disorders [29].

Pharmacological agents of the nonspecific type include amantadine, alpha lipoic acid, buspirone, branched-chain amino acids, creatine, coenzyme Q10, vitamin E, physostigmine, riluzole, and selective serotonin reuptake inhibitors. Specific agents include acetazolamide used for AS2, ACS type 6, and varenicline for spinocerebellar ataxia. Bile acid replacement may be attempted for cerebrotendinous xanthomatosis. Diets such as gluten-free are indicated for gluten ataxia.

Cerebellar tremor may improve with the use of antiepileptic drugs, oscillopsia with memantine and GABA agonists, and spasticity with antispasticity-type medications [30].

A multidisciplinary approach to ataxic disorders may be necessary due to the variability and progressiveness of motor symptoms and non-motor symptoms. Rehabilitation therapies should be offered to all patients with ataxia. Continuous exercise programs have been shown to be effective with positive results [32].

The proposed outline summarizes all potential symptoms clinicians may need to address when facing an ataxic patient. Treatment strategies are often derived from other neurological conditions with similar symptoms and often work. For example, the approach to treating spasticity and bladder symptoms is the same as for people with multiple sclerosis. Assessment and management of these complications are best accomplished with the involvement of therapy specialists, and multidisciplinary teamwork can greatly improve patient care. Carrying out speech therapy is fundamental in the patient's management, including monitoring the swallowing function in the initial stages and seeking to avoid complications while trying to plan nutrition through alternatives such as percutaneous gastrostomy and others (**Figure 1**) [30, 32–34].

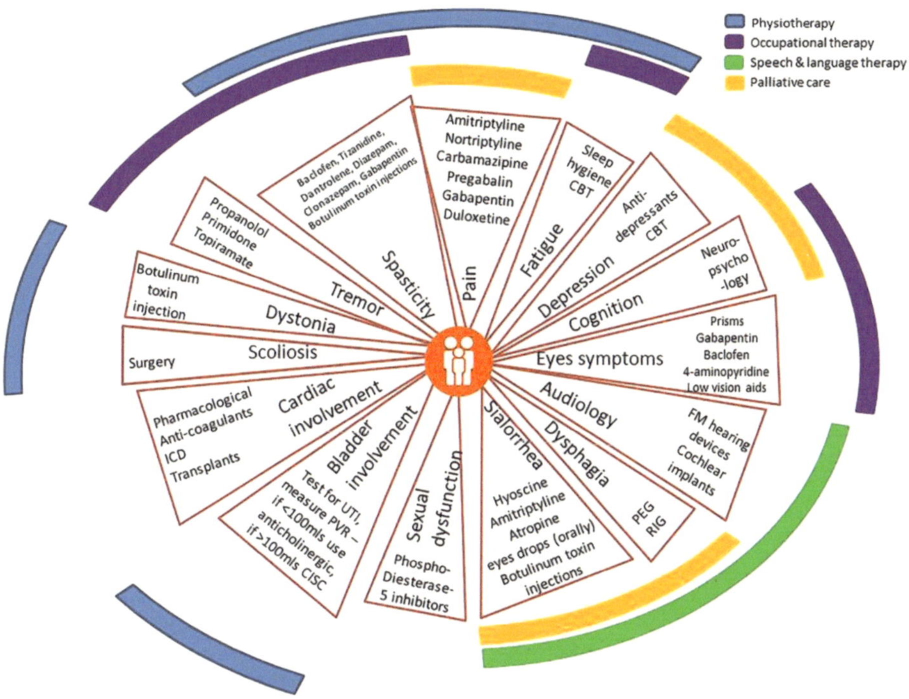

Figure 1.
Common Symptoms of Ataxic Patients and its Treatment Strategies. Extracted from Ref. [9].

8. Final remarks

Due to the very particular nature of ataxia, it is necessary that diagnoses, symptoms or "severity" be evaluated in research targeted at the affected population. It is relevant because, although an intervention may be useful for a population with ataxia who share the same characteristics (e.g., speech problems), it may not be useful without modification for other individuals with other characteristics (e.g., problems that are not problems speech).

To better address the efficacy and safety of treatments for degenerative or hereditary ataxia, longitudinal studies in this field of investigation are also needed. The multidisciplinary team is unquestionably important in the diagnosis and treatment of patients with ataxia. Patients with ataxia typically receive evaluations several times a year, ideally by a specialized team that includes a neurologist, an advanced palliative care nurse, and, as needed, additional medical professionals such as psychiatrists, physiatrists, social workers, palliative, and others.

An important point to remember is that its diagnosis can be more difficult due to the overlapping of phenotypes of different etiologies. Once the common and uncommon presentations of ataxia have been detected, the diagnostic process can be aided by medical history and clinical features, as with any neurological condition. The essential interventions of ataxia disorders can be unraveled through knowledge of the pathophysiological aspects to gain an overview of ataxia along with reading contemporary and up-to-date evidence-based information in various settings. A key point is the correlation of the scenario and age group, identifying whether the disorder appeared in early childhood or even in adulthood and old age. It is the role of an interprofessional team to evaluate the care and management of patients with ataxia, and it is also fundamental, in this case, to take into account the opinions and listen carefully to the patients themselves, caregivers, and professionals involved in forming guidelines for interventions based on their own experiences. The World Health Organization (WHO) highlights September 25 of each year as the international day to raise awareness of these symptoms related to ataxia and this little-known neurological disease, which can sometimes have genetic and hereditary origins.

Finally, future research is imperative to determine whether patients with ataxia can benefit from any type or amount of intervention, according to this review of the intervention domain, as well as improving the ability to detect and differentiate diseases, especially considering that it is a disease, syndrome, and symptom at the same time.

Author details

Caroline Bozzetto Ambrosi[1]* and Patricia Bozzetto Ambrosi[2,3,4,5]*

1 Clinical Medicine and Palliative Care, United Kingdom

2 Independent Clinical Neurology and Imaging Consultant, London, United Kingdom

3 European Academy of Neurology, London, United Kingdom

4 International Association of Hospice and Palliative Care, London, United Kingdom

5 Member of National Ataxia Foundation, London, United Kingdom

*Address all correspondence to: carolboz@gmx.com
and patriciabozzettoadm@outlook.com

References

[1] Hafiz S, De Jesus O. Ataxia. In: StatPearls [Internet]. Treasure Island (FL): StatPearls Publishing; 2023. Available from: https://www.ncbi.nlm.nih.gov/books/NBK562284/ [Accessed: Jun 20, 2023]

[2] Mariotti C, Fancellu R, Di Donato S. An overview of the patient with ataxia. Journal of Neurology. 2005;**252**(5):511-518

[3] Subramony SHA, Durr A. Handbook of clinical neurology. In: (3rd series) Ataxic Disorders Chapter 6- Approach to Ataxic Diseases. Vol. 103. Amsterdam: Elsevier B.V.; 2012. pp. 126-134

[4] National Ataxia Foundation. What is ataxia? [Internet]. 2023 . Available from: https://www.ataxia.org/what-is-ataxia/ [cited November 11 2023] [Accessed: Nov 7, 2023]

[5] Klockgether T. Sporadic ataxia with adult onset: Classification and diagnostic criteria. The Lancet Neurology. 2010;**9**(1):94-104. DOI: 10.1016/S1474-4422(09)70305-9

[6] Perlman S. Hereditary ataxia overview. In: Adam MP, Mirzaa GM, Pagon RA, et al., editors. GeneReviews®. Seattle (WA): University of Washington, Seattle; 1993-2023. Available from: https://www.ncbi.nlm.nih.gov/books/NBK1138/. 1998 Oct 28 [Accessed: Jun 16, 2022]

[7] Brunberg JA. Ataxia. American Journal of Neuroradiology. 2008;**29**(7):1420-1422. Available from: http://www.ajnr.org/content/29/7/1420 [Accessed: October 8, 2023]

[8] Cabaraux P, Gandini J, Manto M. Cerebellum as a CNS hub. Contemporary clinical neuroscience. In: Mizusawa H, Kakei S, editors. The Three Cornerstones of Cerebellar Ataxia: Closing the Loop of 200 Years of Cerebellar Research. Switzerland: Springer; 2021. pp. 459-478

[9] Joyal CC, Meyer C, Jacquart G, Mahler P, Caston J, Lalonde R. Effects of midline and lateral cerebellar lesions on motor coordination and spatial orientation. Brain Research. 1996;**739**(1-2):1-11. DOI: 10.1016/s0006-8993(96)00333-2

[10] Roostaei T, Nazeri A, Sahraian MA, Minagar A. The human cerebellum: A review of physiologic neuroanatomy. Neurologic Clinics. 2014;**32**(4):859-869. DOI: 10.1016/j.ncl.2014.07.013. Epub 2014 Oct 24

[11] Hilger A, Cloud C, Fahey T. Speech impairment in cerebellar ataxia affects naturalness more than intelligibility. Cerebellum. 2023;**22**(4):601-612. DOI: 10.1007/s12311-022-01427-y. Epub 2022 Jun 7

[12] Manto M. The underpinnings of cerebellar ataxias. Clinical Neurophysiology Practice. 2022;**7**: 372-387. DOI: 10.1016/j.cnp.2022.11.002

[13] Schmahmann JD. The cerebellum and cognition. Neuroscience Letters. 2019;**688**:62-75. DOI: 10.1016/j.neulet.2018.07.005. Available from: https://www.sciencedire ct.com/science/article/pii/S0304394018304671

[14] Schmahmann JD. Cognitive and behavioral manifestations of cerebellar strokes: Their relation to motor control and functional topography in the cerebellum. In: Caplan LR, van Gijn J, editors. Stroke Syndromes. 3rd ed. Cambridge UK: Cambridge University Press; 2012. pp. 32-51

[15] Schmahmann JD, MV MM. Cerebellar stroke without motor deficit: Clinical evidence for motor and non-motor domains within the human cerebellum. Neuroscience. 2009;**162**:852-861

[16] Brown S. On hereditary ataxy, with a series of twenty-one cases. Brain. 1892;**15**(2):250-268. DOI: 10.1093/brain/15.2.250

[17] Brusco A, Gellera C, Cagnoli C, Saluto A, Castucci A, Michielotto C, et al. Molecular genetics of hereditary spinocerebellar ataxia: Mutation analysis of spinocerebellar ataxia genes and CAG/CTG repeat expansion detection in 225 Italian families. Archives of Neurology. 2004;**61**:727-733

[18] Stanford Medicine 25. The cerebellar exam [Internet]. Available from: https://stanfordmedicine25.stanford.edu/the25/cerebellar.html. [Accessed: Nov 7, 2023]

[19] National Ataxia Foundation. International Ataxia Awareness Day (IAAD) [Internet]. Available from: https://www.ataxia.org/iaad/ [Accessed: Nov 7, 2023]

[20] Ataxia UK. International Ataxia Awareness Day [Internet]. Available from: https://www.ataxia.org.uk/ataxia-uk-news/international-ataxia-awareness-day/ [Accessed: Nov 7, 2023]

[21] Perez-Lloret S, van de Warrenburg B, Rossi M, Rodríguez-Blázquez C, Zesiewicz T, Saute JAM, et al. Assessment of ataxia rating scales and cerebellar functional tests: Critique and recommendations. Movement Disorders. 2021;**36**:283-297

[22] Schmitz-Hübsch T, Du Montcel ST, Baliko L, Berciano J, Boesch S, Depondt C, et al. Scale for the assessment and rating of ataxia: Development of a new clinical scale. Neurology. 2006;**66**:1717-1720

[23] Trouillas P, Takayanagi T, Hallett M, Currier RD, Subramony SH, Wessel K, et al. International cooperative ataxia rating scale for pharmacological assessment of the cerebellar syndrome. Journal of the Neurological Sciences. 1997;**145**(2):205-211

[24] Subramony SH, May W, Lynch D, Gomez C, Fischbeck K, Hallett M, et al. Measuring Friedreich ataxia: Interrater reliability of a neurologic rating scale. Neurology. 2005;**64**:1261-1262

[25] Meissner WG, Fernagut PO, Dehay B, Péran P, Traon AP-L, Foubert-Samier A, et al. Multiple system atrophy: Recent developments and future perspectives. Movement Disorders. 2019;**34**:1629-1642

[26] Etoom M, Jahan AM, Alghwiri A, Lena F, Modugno N. Ataxia rating scales: Content analysis by linking to the international classification of functioning, disability and health. Healthcare. 2022;**10**(12):2459. DOI: 10.3390/healthcare10122459

[27] Perlman SL. Evaluation and management of ataxia disorders. An overview for physicians. National Ataxia Foundation. 2016:1-20

[28] Khemani P. Overview of Adult-Onset Cerebellar Ataxia, Practical Neurology. 2013. Available from: https://practicalneurology.com/articles/2013-mar-apr/overview-of-adult-onset-cerebellar-ataxia [Accessed: Nov 7, 2023]

[29] Zamora EA, Ahmad T. Dandy-Walker malformation. In: StatPearls. Treasure Island (FL): StatPearls Publishing; 2023. Available from: https://www.ncbi.nlm.nih.gov/books/NBK538197/[Accessed: September 12, 2022]

[30] de Silva RN, Vallortigara J, Greenfield J, et al. Diagnosis and management of progressive ataxia in adults. Practical Neurology. 2019;**19**:196-207

[31] MeSH. Arnold-Chiari malformation [Internet]. Available from: https://meshb.nlm.nih.gov/record/ui?name=Arnold-Chiari+Malformation [Accessed: Nov 7, 2023]

[32] Hadjivassiliou M, Davies-Jones GA, Sanders DS. Dietary treatment of gluten ataxia. Journal of Neurology, Neurosurgery, and Psychiatry. 2003;**74**(9):1221-1224

[33] Fowler CJ, Panicker JN, Drake M, et al. A UK consensus on the management of the bladder in multiple sclerosis. Postgraduate Medical Journal. 2009;**85**:552-559. DOI: 10.1136/jnnp.2008.159178

[34] Logemann JA. Evaluation and Treatment of Swallowing Disorders. Vol. 6. College Hill Press; 1998. pp. 395-400. DOI: 10.1097/00020840-199812000-00008

Section 2

Common Scenarios

Chapter 2

Ataxia Telangiectasia

Barbara Pietrucha

Abstract

Ataxia telangiectasia (AT) is an autosomal recessive disorder characterized by cerebellar degeneration, telangiectasias, immunodeficiency, recurrent sinopulmonary infections, cancer susceptibility, and radiation sensitivity. AT is a complex disorder, whose neurological symptoms most often first appear in early childhood when children begin to sit or walk. They have immunological abnormalities: immunoglobulin and antibody deficiencies and lymphopenia. AT patients have an increased predisposition for cancers, particularly of lymphoid origin. AT is caused by mutations in the *ataxia telangiectasia mutated* (*ATM*) gene, and the role of the ATM protein is the coordination of cellular signaling pathways in response to DNA double-strand breaks, oxidative stress, and other genotoxic stresses. The diagnosis of AT is usually supported by the combination of neurological clinical features and specific laboratory abnormalities (immunoglobulin A (IgA) deficiency, lymphopenia, and increased alpha-fetoprotein (AFP) levels). There are several other neurological and rare disorders that physicians must consider when diagnosing AT. Treatment of neurological symptoms in patients with AT is only symptomatic and supportive, as there are no known treatments that can slow or stop neurodegeneration. However, other symptoms of AT, such as antibody deficiency, lung disease, developmental disorders, diabetes, or cancer, can be effectively treated. Some hope is associated with the treatment of dexamethasone in the patient's own blood cells, which relieves neurological symptoms.

Keywords: ataxia telangiectasia, immunodeficiency, radiation sensitivity, DNA double-strand breaks, ATM protein

1. Introduction

The first description of patients with ataxia telangiectasia (AT) was published in 1926 [1], but it was not until 1958 that the term "ataxia telangiectasia" was first coined. AT was given its commonly used name by Elena Boder and Robert P. Sedgwick, who described a familial syndrome of progressive cerebellar ataxia, oculocutaneous telangiectasia, and frequent pulmonary infection [2]. Ataxia telangiectasia, or AT, is also referred to as the Louis-Bar syndrome (OMIM #208900). Orphanet Orpha Number: ORPHA100.

Ataxia telangiectasia is an autosomal recessive cerebellar ataxia [3]. It is also included in inborn errors of immunity (IEI) with chromosomal instability, DNA repair disorders, and less commonly known as neurocutaneous syndrome [4]. The disease is caused by a mutation in the *ataxia telangiectasia mutated* (*ATM*) gene encoding the serine-threonine protein kinase [5, 6]. ATM is a large protein

(~350 kDa) with a critical role in DNA double-strand break (DSB) repair, genome stability, cell cycle regulation, and cell survival [7]. The ATM protein is involved in natural physiological processes during DNA replication, meiosis, mitosis, V (variable), D (diversity), or J (joining) recombination or immunoglobulin class switching (CSR, class switch recombination). In addition, other targets of the ATM protein are those involved in oxidative stress metabolism [8]. ATM is mainly a nuclear protein, but it is also found in the cytoplasm and regulates the function of mitochondria and peroxisomes, and through this it affects angiogenesis and glucose metabolism. Lack of ATM protein function is associated with the development of certain disorders in AT patients, such as progressive neurodegeneration, immune deficiencies, pulmonary, metabolic, dermatological, and vascular complications [9–11].

Ataxia telangiectasia is characterized by progressive cerebellar degeneration, oculocutaneous telangiectasias, immunodeficiency, recurrent sinopulmonary infections, radiation sensitivity, premature aging, and susceptibility to cancer development, especially of lymphoid origin. Other abnormalities, such as growth failure, poor pubertal development, gonadal atrophy, insulin-resistant diabetes, lung diseases, cutaneous abnormality, and cardiovascular disease, have also been reported in AT patients [12–14].

The prevalence of AT is estimated to be <1–9/100,000. However, the incidence of AT may be higher 1/40,000 in consanguineous population or those populations with founder effect [15]. AT patients have poor prognosis; the median survival is 25 years with a wide range. The two most common causes of death in these patients are chronic pulmonary diseases and malignancy [14, 16]. AT patients show remarkable clinical and laboratory differences that reflect the presence of genotype/phenotype correlations in these patients or other genetic/environmental disease-modifying factors. The majority of ATM mutations lead to a truncated protein, while some missense and splicing site variations cause milder phenotype [17].

Ataxia telangiectasia patients have much milder clinical progress as a result of retained expression of either normal [18, 19] or mutant ATM protein with residual activity [20–22]. These patients often retain the ability to walk into adulthood and consequently might be diagnosed when adults [19, 23]. The terms "classic" and "mild" are used to distinguish two different but widely recognized clinical presentations of AT. People with mild AT have less severe, later onset of symptoms associated with longer survival. Ataxia telangiectasia-like disorder (ATLD) [24–26], ataxia oculomotor apraxia type 1 (AOA1) [27, 28], and ataxia oculomotor apraxia type 2 (AOA2) [29–32] have neurological features similar to those of AT.

2. Clinical picture and management

In the classic presentation of AT, ataxia is often the first diagnostic sign that appears during the toddler years, usually manifest between 6 and 18 months of age. Children also have difficulty standing or sitting still and may sway slowly side-to-side or backwards. Because most of the children with classic AT have stable neurological symptoms for the first 4–5 years of life, they can initially be diagnosed as having "ataxic cerebral palsy" [33]. Beyond the age of 10, the movement problems typically cause a child to be confined to a wheelchair [34]. Eye movement abnormalities emerge in early school years. Dysarthria, which is the consequence of impaired coordination of respiratory, phonatory, and bulbar functions, can occur at any time and may or may not progress [35, 36]. Drooling may persist beyond expected ages. Swallowing difficulties typically worsen in early teen years. Most of these neurological problems stop progressing after the age of about 12–15 years. AT patients manifest hallmarks of cerebellar dysfunction such as truncal swaying, gait ataxia, dyssynergia, muscle hypotonia, and sudden falls [33], and may have abnormal involuntary movements, including chorea, dystonia, dysphagia, athetosis, myoclonic jerks, or various tremors [37, 38]. Other extrapyramidal symptoms may include body hypokinesia or bradykinesia and facial hypomimia [34, 35]. Distal-to-proximal advancing loss of tendon reflexes is also characteristic of AT [39], reflecting a progressive sensory and motor neuropathy [35, 40].

Cerebellar degeneration in AT originates from atrophy of cerebellar vermis and hemispheres involving the dendrites and axons of Purkinje cells (PCs) and granule neurons [2]. However, microcephaly does not usually occur in AT patients because it is caused by the progressive accelerated aging process. For the majority of AT patients, neuroimaging studies in the toddler years and early childhood years are normal. As the disease progresses, MRI studies support the pathological finding of progressive and diffuse cerebellar atrophy [34, 41]. Due to the radiation exposure inherent in computed tomography (CT), MRI is the preferred method of visualizing the central nervous system (CNS) in patients with AT. Intellectual disability is not a common sign in AT; however, it occasionally occurs [8]. The correlation of neurodegenerative phenotype and ATM deficiency remains unclear, but the hypothesis suggested that ATM is the main player in maintaining cellular homeostasis and preventing disease in the nervous system. The prevailing dogma in the field is that specific neuronal cells within the cerebellum (primarily Purkinje and granule cells) are particularly sensitive to the loss of ATM. Normal ATM protein may allow neurons to repair damage DNA or initiate apoptotic pathway [42, 43]. On the other hand, neurodegeneration may be attributable to deficient-reactive oxygen species (ROS) homeostasis following dysfunction of ATM in neurons [34].

The second major symptom of AT ocular telangiectasias often occurs after the onset of neurological symptoms, usually by the age of 5–8 years, sometimes later or never. The absence of telangiectasias does not exclude the diagnosis, but is a common cause of delayed diagnosis [44, 45]. Telangiectasias may also appear on sun-exposed areas of skin in some patients and in other locations such as the pharyngeal wall, and have been seen deep inside the brain of older people with AT. The ocular telangiectasia do not bleed or itch, though they are sometimes misdiagnosed due to chronic conjunctivitis or allergy [20, 46].

Other ocular symptoms include: abnormal eye movement and visual disturbances caused by degeneration of the cerebellar cortex manifesting in AT including oculomotor apraxia, periodic alternating nystagmus (PAN), gaze-evoked nystagmus, strabismus, and vestibulo-ocular (VOR) abnormalities [47–49]. Patients with AT have prominent defects in the eye movement systems that stabilize images on the retina and in the systems that shift direction of gaze.

The next clinical manifestation of AT are recurrent respiratory infections. Chronic lung disease develops in more than 25% of people with AT, mostly progressing with the increasing age and neurological deterioration. Respiratory complications are the leading cause of morbidity and mortality among AT patients, as 50% of patients die in adolescence from respiratory failure [13, 16, 50]. Generally, there are three major types of lung diseases in AT patients, including recurrent sinopulmonary infections and bronchiectasis, interstitial lung disease (ILD)/pulmonary fibrosis, and neuromuscular disorders affecting respiratory function [13, 51, 52]. The pathogenesis of lung disease in AT patients is multifactorial, related to immune deficiency, abnormal

DNA damage repair, signs of premature aging, chronic inflammation, and oxidative stress [53]. Patients with respiratory infections are most often found to have reduced or absent serum immunoglobulin G2 (IgG2) and a defect in class switch recombination (CSR) [54, 55]. These mechanisms are associated with disease progression due to recurrent infections, emphysema, ineffective cough and airway clearance disorders, and oropharyngeal dysphagia [51, 52, 56].

People with AT have a decrease in their measured forced vital capacity (FVC). This may result in a functionally restrictive lung phenotype, similar to that with neuromuscular weakness associated with reduced lung reserve. A weak or ineffective cough leading to impaired mucociliary clearance (MCC) can also contribute to reduced respiratory capacity. Reduced FVC and MCC can cause recurrent respiratory infections. In addition, the situation is exacerbated by the presence of immunodeficiencies, aspiration, increased chromosomal breakage, cell senescence, inflammation, and impaired DNA damage repair due to ATM deficiency [56–58]. Shortened telomeres and sensitivity to ionizing radiation are also characteristic of AT and can increase the risk of complications such as pulmonary fibrosis when treating malignancies [59, 60].

Interstitial lung disease has been described in individuals with AT, although the exact incidence is unknown. In patients with AT who died from chronic respiratory disease, ILD was present in about 25% [61]. Symptoms of ILD include a nonproductive cough lasting >1 month, shortness of breath, and fever. There are abnormal auscultatory changes over the lungs, and interstitial changes on chest radiography. ILD can occur even in the absence of immunodeficiency. Antibiotic therapy does not result in improvement [62]. Diagnosis of ILD on the basis of clinical examination is often difficult because symptoms are nonspecific. Restrictive lung disease on pulmonary function testing may suggest the presence of an interstitial process. In AT patients with pulmonary symptoms that do not completely resolve after intensive treatment of the infection, chest radiography is helpful, but due to increased radiosensitivity, MRI may become the technique of choice. A lung biopsy is required to confirm the diagnosis of ILD. However, the diagnostic benefits of a procedure such as a lung biopsy should always be weighed against the risks associated with anesthesia and surgery [62]. It should be considered that in patients with AT, secondary pulmonary lymphoma may clinically and radiographically mimic ILD [63]. The increased risk of developing pulmonary fibrosis in patients with AT may be a result of chemotherapy for malignancies [60]. In patients with AT, progressive neuromuscular decline can worsen pulmonary function, e.g., bulbar muscle dysfunction can result in swallowing dysfunction and chronic aspiration [13, 57].

Chronic lung disease is the leading cause of death in AT (about 30%), and early intervention is key to preventing or slowing its progression. Pulmonary function tests should be performed in all children with AT starting at the age of 6 and continued annually [56, 64], and performed prior to any surgical procedure requiring anesthesia.

Chest computed tomography (CT), considered to be the "gold standard," is the best tool for assessing changes in chronic lung disease (CLD) [65]. Due to hypersensitivity to radiation, exposure to ionizing radiation should be avoided in patients with AT [66, 67]. MRI of the chest becomes such a method, which is a useful nonradiation tool in several lung diseases, because it is highly compatible with computed tomography of the chest [68–70].

The manifestation of immunodeficiency in AT is usually sinopulmonary infections that are often manifested early in life [13, 51]. Abnormalities of the immune system are observed in approximately two-thirds of patients with AT due to impaired antigen receptor recombination and class switch recombination (CSR). Generally, selective immunoglobulin A (IgA) deficiency, hypogammaglobulinemia, immunoglobulin G (IgG) subclasses' deficiency, gammopathy, and failure to make specific antibodies in responses to vaccines or infections are frequent findings in AT patients [71, 72]. A small percentage of patients with AT may also have hyper-immunoglobulin M (hyper-IgM). Since some existing symptoms of AT, such as atactic gait and dysarthria, might not be present in infancy, the diagnosis of these patients may be confused with the diagnosis of hyper-IgM syndrome [73–75]. The most common deficiencies of cellular immunity are lymphopenia with decreased B- and T cells, reduced number and faulty functioning of CD4+ T lymphocytes [71, 76]. The progressive reduction of the cellular compartment during life may reduce life expectancy of people with AT [77]. Another problem in AT patients is an increased risk of developing autoimmune and/or chronic inflammatory diseases that are associated with immune dysregulation [78, 79]. About a quarter of patients with AT may have autoimmune disorder, the most frequent organ involved being the skin with vitiligo and psoriasis. Diseases, such as Hashimoto's thyroiditis (HT), juvenile idiopathic arthritis (JIA), immune thrombocytopenic purpura (ITP), and autoimmune hemolytic anemia (AIHA), have also been reported [80–82].

All patients with AT should have at least one comprehensive immunological evaluation to assess the number and type of B- and T cells, the levels of serum immunoglobulins (IgG, IgM, and IgA) and antibody responses to T cell-dependent (e.g., tetanus, *Hemophilus influenzae* b) and T cell-independent (pneumococcal polysaccharide) vaccines [51, 83].

There are no general recommendations as to how often immunological tests should be repeated, certainly they should be performed when problems with infections occur or worsen [56, 84, 85].

Immunization of people with AT may be less effective, and these individuals often have a suboptimal response to pneumococcal vaccine, as well as to other vaccines [86]. If antibody function is normal, all routine childhood immunizations should be given, except the measles, mumps and rubella (MMR) vaccine [56]. Among other reasons, because chronic cutaneous granulomas can be associated with AT [87, 88] and they have been linked to replication of the incompetent rubella virus vaccine strain detected by PCR [89–91].

There are also skin lesions. Common skin abnormalities associated with AT include oculocutaneous telangiectasias, skin atrophy, café-au-lait spots, vitiligo, seborrheic dermatitis, and premature graying [92–94]. These patients may also have an increased incidence of vitiligo and warts, which may be due to immunodeficiency, making treatment of these complications difficult [51]. Other skin changes are cutaneous granulomas with unknown pathogenesis that occur uncommonly in various inborn errors of immunity (IEI) and manifest in almost 10% of AT patients [95]. These lesions have not been associated with an identifiable pathogen, but sometimes can be associated with painful ulceration, bleeding, or might erode down to muscle or bone [87, 96].

It has been proposed that cutaneous granulomas can be considered as a manifestation of dysregulation in innate immunity, wound healing, and tissue repair explained by the immune defects in these primary immunodeficiency disorders (PIDs) [87]. Recent data suggest that more than 40% of AT patients with cutaneous granulomas present a hyper-IgM phenotype. AT patients with granulomas had an equal distribution of all lymphocyte subsets, except for a significant reduction in B cells, naive CD4+ cells and naive CD8+ T cells, in the presence of normal total natural killer (NK) and T cells [11, 87]. B cells, CD19+, appear to play a fundamental role in wound healing; it was observed that mouse CD19 deficiency stopped skin wound healing [97].

Recently, an association has been found between the administration of live rubella vaccines and the formation of cutaneous and visceral rubella-positive granulomatous in people with AT, as well as in other immunodeficiencies with impaired DNA repair [98, 99].

Poor growth is a common feature in classic AT [100–102]. Various factors may influence growth failure in AT. They include chronic infections, insulin-like growth factor 1 (IGF-1) hormone deficiency, and reduced nutrient intake due to fatigue and swallowing problems [84, 102–104]. On the other hand, growth retardation is common in patients with AT and may be a primary feature of the disease, directly related to the ATM mutation. The study, in an Israeli cohort of patients with AT, demonstrated that impaired growth was more prominent in females than males, and that this difference is apparent at an age before gonadotropins begin to affect growth rates. Delayed pubertal development is often described as an aspect of AT. Gonadal atrophy or dysgenesis resulting in delayed pubertal development and early menopause has been reported [105–107]. We know of pregnancies in people with mild AT, but not in anyone with the classic form of the disease [108 and own observations].

Vitamin D deficiency has been commonly found in patients with AT, given the implications for bone health and possibly for susceptibility to malignancies [12].

People with AT have been found to have cholesterol profiles associated with a higher risk for cardiovascular disease [109], diabetes with insulin resistance [110], and steatohepatitis [111, 112]. These findings suggest that ATM dysregulation is associated with the development of metabolic syndrome, demonstrating a significant role of functional protein in glucose and insulin metabolism [113, 114]. People with AT should undergo screening for these conditions during adolescence and early adult life so that timely treatments can be initiated.

People with AT have an increased predisposition to malignancy, ranging from 10 to 25% [73, 115]. The most common types of malignancies in patients with AT are lymphoid tumor. Leukemias and lymphomas (T-cell acute lymphoblastic leukemias [ALLs] and T-cell lymphocytic leukemias [T-PLL]) tend to occur in younger patients under the age of 20. These two types of cancers account for 85% of all malignancies in children [116]. B-cell non-Hodgkin's lymphoma (NHL) and Hodgkin's lymphoma (HL) have also been frequently described in patients with AT [117, 118]. Adult patients with AT are susceptible to both lymphoid malignancies and solid tumors, such as cancers of the breast, stomach, liver, parotid gland, and esophagus [84, 119].

Another factor that may predispose to the development of lymphomas (such as HL and B-cell NHL) is the Epstein-Barr virus (EBV). Individuals with AT present an impaired immune response to EBV infection, which is associated with cellular immune deficiencies and DNA repair defects [11, 120].

Adults with AT may benefit from annual whole-body MRIs to screen for malignancies. Patients diagnosed with malignancy should be treated in specialist centers and treatment modifications and dose reductions are usually needed to minimize side effects and optimize outcomes [121, 122].

Heterozygous carriers of the ATM mutation have an increased risk of developing breast cancer, with an estimated risk of 5.1 over that in the whole population, whereas there is no evidence for an increased risk of lymphoid malignancies [119, 123]. A 2016 meta-analysis found the cumulative risk of breast cancer in carriers to amount to approximately 6% by age 50 and 30% by age 80 [124]. While there is insufficient evidence that ATM heterozygotes may increase the risk of other cancers, there are studies suggesting an increased risk of gastric and colorectal cancers [125]. Cancer screening guidelines are being developed for ATM mutation carriers. Standard breast cancer surveillance, including monthly breast self-exam, yearly breast MRI and mammogram and, additionally for both male and female ATM mutation carriers, colon cancer screenings with a colonoscopy (every 3–5 years compared to every 10 years for the whole of the population), should be performed [126].

Another complication observed in older people with AT pertains to orthopedic complications: these include an acquired clubfoot deformity and, less commonly, scoliosis. Sometimes finger contractures develop, most often due to inflammatory connective tissue disease, but sometimes due to neuropathy [127 and own observation].

Some people with AT suffer from bladder and/or bowel incontinence, recurrent vomiting especially in the morning, decreased sleep efficiency, and dizziness which may connect with neurological complications [84, 128].

Feeding and swallowing (chewing) can become difficult for people with AT as they get older [52]. Involuntary movements can make it difficult to eat independently and cause a mess or extend meal times excessively. Dysphagia is common in AT and usually appears in the second decade of life due to neurological changes that impair the coordination of oropharyngeal movements. Problems involving the pharynx can cause aspiration of fluids, food, and saliva. Dysphagia with silent aspiration can cause pulmonary sequelae in AT [52].

Dysphagia can also cause nutritional deficiencies, as the process of eating becomes slow and difficult. Some people with AT stop eating or reduce their food intake due to frustration or fatigue with the process. Inadequate caloric intake can contribute to stunted growth in children and weight maintenance in the elderly, causing a lower body mass index (BMI) compared to healthy, age-matched controls [104, 129–131]. Poor nutrition can exacerbate symptoms of neurological disability. Abnormal respiratory-swallowing coupling is associated with an increased risk of aspiration and can cause swallowing problems before the development of feeding and pulmonary sequelae in AT [132].

3. AT diagnosis

A clinical diagnosis of AT can usually be made on the basis of the presence of characteristic neurological and non-neurological clinical signs and specific laboratory findings. Laboratory studies may be helpful in diagnosing AT by finding elevated alpha-fetoprotein (AFP) levels after age 1, spontaneous and X-ray-induced chromosomal breaks and/or rearrangements in cultured lymphoblastoid cell lines, and reduced cell survival after irradiation [133]. Imaging studies show cerebellar atrophy, not always apparent on MRI in young children, which does not necessarily correlate with the clinical picture [127].

The most common immunological abnormalities found in AT are deficiency of serum IgA, IgE, and selective IgG subscales, elevated IgM levels, lymphopenia (affecting mainly T lymphocytes), and reduced diversity of the T-cell receptor (TCR) immune repertoire [51, 71]. It is important to combine the symptoms present with the results of laboratory tests. A definitive diagnosis can be confirmed by the absence or deficiency of ATM kinase activity, measured in a lymphoblastoid cell line derived from the patient's blood or in fibroblasts from a skin biopsy, and finally the detection of pathological mutations in the *ATM* gene. As elevated serum AFP levels are observed in ≥95% of patients with AT and these levels should therefore be assessed in any child >1 year of age with unexplained atactic gait [134, 135]. The cause of elevated

Disorder	Gene	Ataxia	Telangiectasia	Immunodeficiency	Radiosensitivity	Malignancy	AFP
A-T	*ATM*	+	+	+	+	+	↑
ATLD1	*MRE11*	+	—	—	+	NK	N
ATLD2	*PCNA*	+	+	—	NK	+	N
AOA1	*APTX*	+	—	—	+	—	N
AOA2	*SETX*	+	—	—	—	—	↑
NBS	*NBS1*	—	—	+	+	++	N
RIDDLE	*RNF168*	+/–	+	+	+	NK	↑

ataxia-telangiectasia (A-T), ATLD 1 – ataxia telangiectasia-like disorder 1 (ATLD1), ataxia telangiectasia-like disorder 2 (ATLD2), ataxia oculomotor apraxia type 1 (AOA1), ataxia oculomotor apraxia type 2 (AOA2), Nijmegen breakage syndrome (NBS), radiosensitivity, immunodeficiency, dysmorphic features, and learning difficulties (RIDDLE), alpha-fetoprotein (AFP).

Table 1.
Clinical and laboratory features of rare genetic disorders that can be discriminate with A-T.

serum AFP levels in most people with AT remains unknown. Assessment of AFP levels can be a helpful tool in the early diagnosis of AT [45].

As the whole exome sequencing becomes increasingly standard clinical practice for individuals with unusual and/or unexplained symptoms, it is likely that more people with mild forms of AT will be diagnosed [136]. This will necessarily change our views on the phenotypic expression of AT. Prenatal genetic diagnosis is possible when prospective parents each have confirmed pathogenetic mutations in ATM. Preimplantation genetic diagnosis (PGD) can avoid the birth of an affected child in parents who have an affected child (or children) with AT. At least two such cases have been described in the literature so far [137, 138].

Additionally, the newborn screening (NBS) test for severe combined immunodeficiency (SCID), introduced in recent years, can identify children born with other immunodeficiencies, including AT, which involve a deficiency or absence of T and B lymphocytes [139, 140]. Despite the lack of effective treatments for AT, early diagnosis allows for genetic counseling and family education, as well as intensive supportive care. Genetic counseling can provide AT genetic testing for siblings and other family members and help interpret test results.

Differential diagnosis. There are some rare disorders that can be misdiagnosis with AT based on similar clinical and laboratory features. The most common disorders that are sometimes confused with AT are: cerebral palsy (CP) and Friedreich's ataxia (FA or FRDA). Each of these diseases can be distinguished from AT based on neurological examination and clinical history. CP, unlike AT, is a nonprogressive motor dysfunction resulting from early brain injury [141]. In addition, most children with CP manifest regional or diffuse spasticity in a pattern not seen in AT. Children with ataxia due to CP will not manifest laboratory abnormalities associated with AT. In FRDA, symptoms usually tend to present later between the ages of 10 and 16 and differ from AT in the absence of telangiectasias and oculomotor apraxia, the early absence of tendon reflexes, a normal AFP, the frequent presence of scoliosis, cardiomyopathy, and abnormal ECG features [84, 142].

Other disorders with childhood-onset ataxia include ataxia telangiectasia like disorder 2 (ATLD2), ataxia oculomotor apraxia type 1 (AOA1), ataxia oculomotor apraxia type 2 (AOA2), radiosensitivity, immunodeficiency, dysmorphic features, and learning difficulties (RIDDLE) syndrome (RNF168 deficiency), and spinocerebellar ataxia with axonal neuropathy (SCAN1).

Immunodeficiency is one of the common symptoms of Nijmegen breakage syndrome (NBS, with birds like face and microcephaly), ataxia telangiectasia like disorder 1 (ATLD1, due to meiotic recombination 11 homolog A (MRE11) deficiency), and RIDDLE syndrome that can be confused with AT. As in AT, elevated serum AFP levels are also present in AOA2 and RIDDLE syndrome. Therefore, knowledge of the gene mutation in a child with ataxia, immunodeficiency, telangiectasias, radiosensitivity, and elevated AFP can distinguish AT from other disorders with ataxia of childhood onset [11, 143]. A comparison of the clinical and laboratory features of these disorders is shown in **Table 1**.

4. AT treatment

Treatment of AT is symptomatic and supportive. As regards the neurological symptoms, no therapy can slow degeneration, but physical, occupational, and speech therapies as well as exercise may help maintain function. In some patients, certain anti-Parkinson and antiepileptic drugs may partially ameliorate symptoms. Commonly prescribed drugs include trihexyphenidyl (an antimuscarinic), amantadine (an antiparkinsonian) [144], baclofen (an antispastic), and botulinum toxin injections (a paralytic). Less commonly used drugs that may also be beneficial include gabapentin and pregabalin (an anticonvulsant), and clonazepam (a tranquilizer and antiseizure medication) [34, 145]. Also, glucocorticoids (especially betamethasone) have been reported to improve neurological symptoms in AT but corticosteroid side effects were quickly observed [146]. To avoid the characteristic side effects of long-term steroid administration, a method of monthly infusions of autologous erythrocytes loaded with dexamethasone has been developed (EryDex; EryDel, Urbino, Italy). Preliminary results are promising, with demonstrated efficacy in improving neurological status, especially in young patients with AT [147, 148].

Regular screening to assess lung function can detect early deterioration of lung function and allow earlier intervention. These interventions may include chest physiotherapy, a cough support device, and assistance to improve MCC. These interventions can be used daily as maintenance therapies. In some children with AT, with bronchial hyperresponsiveness, bronchodilators may benefit [57]. Children with chronic or recurrent sinopulmonary disease should be treated with antibiotics when appropriate, chest physiotherapy and airway clearance techniques to reduce the risk of developing bronchiectasis and chronic lung disease [57].

To maintain respiratory muscle strength and minimize the progression of lung disease, it is important to have adequate nutrition and maintain a normal body mass index. All people with AT should avoid secondhand smoke exposure and have minimal exposure to other environmental pollution. If lung disease develops, appropriate management should be considered: liberal use of antibiotics, antibiotic prophylaxis, corticosteroids, and immunoglobulin supplementation in those patients with AT who are immunocompromised [57, 62].

Recurrent lung infections may involve dysfunctional swallow (dysphagia) with aspiration, but some people with AT can be taught to drink, chew, and swallow more safely reducing the risk of aspiration [56]. Because the nutritional deficit in some people with AT may be more severe than previously appreciated, early nutritional intervention and ongoing nutritional support and education for patients, families, and caregivers are crucial [101, 149].

High-calorie foods are then recommended, and a gastrostomy tube (G-tube or feeding tube) is rarely used. A gastrostomy tube is recommended when a child cannot eat enough to grow, is not gaining weight and when dysphagia with aspiration causes breathing problems and/or when meals take too long or stressful [150].

People with IgG deficiency or impaired antibody function should receive standard immunoglobulin replacement therapy. Despite the low T-lymphocyte count found, prophylactic antibiotic use to prevent opportunistic infections is not necessary, unless individuals are treated chronically with corticosteroids, other immunosuppressive drugs, or chemotherapy [56, 84, 85]. Individuals with normal ability to produce antibody should receive an annual influenza vaccine, and additional pneumococcal vaccines at intervals to maintain high levels of antipneumococcal antibodies [85].

Cutaneous granulomas can be persistent, progressive, and very difficult to treat. To date, treatment has been attempted with topical and systemic corticosteroids, intravenous immunoglobulin, antitumor necrosis factor therapy, and antiviral therapy, with either mediocre or transient results [96, 151]. Only in immunodeficient patients with DNA repair disorders who underwent hematopoietic stem cell transplantation due to cancer observed granuloma healing [152, 153, and own observation].

In adolescent females, sex hormone replacement therapy may need to be considered to support optimal linear growth, development of secondary sex symptoms, and prevention of osteoporosis. Vitamin D levels should be monitored and treated with an appropriate dose [12].

Despite the poor prognosis of many AT cancers, they manage to be successfully treated. Cancer treatment should only take place in specialized oncology centers and only after consultation with a clinician who has specific experience in AT. Standard cancer treatment regimens should be modified to minimize or prevent cytotoxicity from radiomimetic drugs [73, 85]. Radiotherapy can only be used exceptionally and at reduced doses. The use of cyclophosphamide needs to be monitored as late onset of severe hemorrhage from bladder telangiectasia has been observed [154]. Even with modified therapy, late complications of chemotherapy are observed in some people with AT [155]. Although routine bone marrow transplantation is not currently recommended [156], it has however been performed successfully in several cases of hematopoietic malignancies in AT [157, 158].

5. Quality of life

Children with AT experience varying degrees of difficulty in functioning at school due to progressive neurodegeneration. There is an impairment of fine and gross motor coordination, resulting in reduced writing and computer skills. Dysarthria and delayed speech initiation, poor facial expressions, and delayed reaction time to visual and verbal cues, which limit the ability to communicate, are observed. Eye movement disorders with oculomotor apraxia limit reading ability. Mental and physical fatigue is commonly observed. People with AT, through the prism of motor disability, may additionally be perceived as intellectually impaired without actually having any impairment. Social awareness is usually normal. Although this disparity can lead to social isolation and depression, many people with AT do well to overcome these difficulties, especially in the presence of a supportive environment at school. As survival and quality of life improve, some people with AT manage to complete higher education and lead independent lives with support [85].

6. Final remarks

That's why a number of voluntary patient organizations and support groups have sprung up in various countries around the world, working closely with scientific and medical experts to find effective therapies to improve quality of life and provide education and support for families affected by AT. The most active internationally are the AT Children's Project from the USA and the AT Society from the UK. In October 2014, a clinical guidance document on the diagnosis and treatment of ataxia telangiectasia in children was published by the UK AT Society [128]. To quickly make data on people with AT available to researchers and doctors for analysis, the Global AT Family Data Platform was launched in July 2016 [159]. In parallel with the Platform and voluntary patient organizations, work is underway on an international registry of patients with AT. The registry will include baseline and longitudinal data provided by clinicians and clinical centers that treat people with AT. Analysis of data from growing patient registries [128, 159] will inform natural history, improve disease management, and aid therapy development.

7. Conclusion

1. There are still many unresolved questions regarding the complexity and severity of AT, such as the influence of environmental factors, disease-modifying genes, epigenetics, telomere length, and the gut microbiome on the presentation, severity, and progression of various AT manifestations, which remain unknown.

2. Researchers are investigating ways to apply recent breakthroughs in the fields of gene and mutation-targeted therapies to AT [160, 161].

Author details

Barbara Pietrucha
Department of Immunology, The Children's Memorial Health Institute, Warsaw, Poland

*Address all correspondence to: barbara.p@rocketmail.com

References

[1] Henner K. Apropos of the description of "ataxia teleangiectasis" by Mme Louis-Bar. Priority of the description, by lad. Syllaba and K. Henner in 1926, of the conjunctival vascular network. Revue Neurologique (Paris). 1968;**118**(1):60-63

[2] Boder E, Sedgwik RP. Ataxia-telangiectasia; a familial syndrome of progressive cerebellar ataxia, oculocutaneous telangiectasia and frequent pulmonary infection. Pediatrics. 1958;**21**(4):526-554

[3] Anheim M, Tranchant C, Koenig M. The autosomal recessive cerebellar ataxias. The New England Journal of Medicine. 2012;**366**(7):636-646

[4] Tangye SG, Al-Herz W, Bousfiha A, Cunningham-Rundles C, Franco JL, Holland SM, et al. Human inborn errors of immunity: 2022 update on the classification from the International Union of Immunological Societies Expert Committee. Journal of Clinical Immunology. 2022;**42**(7):1473-1507

[5] Gatti RA, Berkel I, Boder E, Braedt G, Charmley P, Concannon P, et al. Localization of an ataxia-telangiectasia gene to chromosome 11q22-23. Nature. 1988;**336**(6199):577-580

[6] Savitsky K, Bar-Shira A, Gilad S, Rotman G, Ziv Y, Vanagaite L, et al. A single ataxia telangiectasia gene with a product similar to PI-3 kinase. Science. 1995;**268**(5218):1749-1753

[7] Lavin MF, Gueven N, Grattan-Smith P. Defective responses to DNA single- and double-strand breaks in spinocerebellar ataxia. DNA Repair (Amst). 2008;**7**(7):1061-1076

[8] Chun HH, Gatti RA. Ataxia-telangiectasia, an evolving phenotype. DNA Repair (Amst). 2004;**3**(8-9):1187-1196

[9] Ambrose M, Goldstine JV, Gatti RA. Intrinsic mitochondrial dysfunction in ATM-deficient lymphoblastoid cells. Human Molecular Genetics. 2007;**16**(18):2154-2164

[10] Valentin-Vega YA, Maclean KH, Tait-Mulder J, Milasta S, Steeves M, Dorsey FC, et al. Mitochondrial dysfunction in ataxia-telangiectasia. Blood. 2012;**119**(6):1490-1500

[11] Amirifar P, Ranjouri MR, Yazdani R, Abolhassani H, Aghamohammadi A. Ataxia-telangiectasia: A review of clinical features and molecular pathology. Pediatric Allergy and Immunology. 2019;**30**(3):277-288

[12] Nissenkorn A, Levy-Shraga Y, Banet-Levi Y, Lahad A, Sarouk I, Modan-Moses D. Endocrine abnormalities in ataxia telangiectasia: Findings from a national cohort. Pediatric Research. 2016;**79**(6):889-894

[13] Bott L, Lebreton J, Thumerelle C, Cuvellier J, Deschildre A, Sardet A. Lung disease in ataxia-telangiectasia. Acta Paediatrica. 2007;**96**(7):1021-1024

[14] Su Y, Swift M. Mortality rates among carriers of ataxia-telangiectasia mutant alleles. Annals of Internal Medicine. 2000;**133**(10):770-778

[15] Swift M, Morrell D, Cromartie E, Chamberlin AR, Skolnick MH, Bishop DT. The incidence and gene frequency of ataxia-telangiectasia in the United States. American Journal of Human Genetics. 1986;**39**(5):573-583

[16] Crawford TO, Skolasky RL, Fernandez R, Rosquist KJ,

Lederman HM. Survival probability in ataxia telangiectasia. Archives of Disease in Childhood. 2006;**91**(7):610-611

[17] Gilad S, Chessa L, Khosravi R, Russell P, Galanty Y, Piane M, et al. Genotype-phenotype relationships in ataxia-telangiectasia and variants. American Journal of Human Genetics. 1998;**62**(3):551-561

[18] McConville CM, Stankovic T, Byrd PJ, McGuire GM, Yao QY, Lennox GG, et al. Mutations associated with variant phenotypes in ataxia-telangiectasia. American Journal of Human Genetics. 1996;**59**(2):320-330

[19] Sutton IJ, Last JI, Ritchie SJ, Harrington HJ, Byrd PJ, Taylor AM. Adult-onset ataxia telangiectasia due to ATM 5762ins137 mutation homozygosity. Annals of Neurology. 2004;**55**(6):891-895

[20] Carrillo F, Schneider SA, Taylor AM, Srinivasan V, Kapoor R, Bhatia KP. Prominent oromandibular dystonia and pharyngeal telangiectasia in atypical ataxia telangiectasia. Cerebellum. 2009;**8**(1):22-27

[21] Verhagen MM, Abdo WF, Willemsen MA, Hogervorst FB, Smeets DF, Hiel JA, et al. Clinical spectrum of ataxia-telangiectasia in adulthood. Neurology. 2009;**73**(6):430-437

[22] Stewart GS, Last JI, Stankovic T, Haites N, Kidd AM, Byrd PJ, et al. Residual ataxia telangiectasia mutated protein function in cells from ataxia telangiectasia patients, with 5762ins137 and 7271T-->G mutations, showing a less severe phenotype. The Journal of Biological Chemistry. 2001;**276**(32):30133-30141

[23] Hiel JAP, van Engelen BGM, Weemaes CMR, Broeks A, Verrips A, ter Laak H, et al. Distal spinal muscular atrophy as a major feature in adult-onset ataxia telangiectasia. Neurology. 2006;**67**(2):346-349

[24] Stewart GS, Maser RS, Stankovic T, Bressan DA, Kaplan MI, Jaspers NG, et al. The DNA double-strand break repair gene hMRE11 is mutated in individuals with an ataxia-telangiectasia-like disorder. Cell. 1999;**99**(6):577-587

[25] Delia D, Piane M, Buscemi G, Savio C, Palmeri S, Lulli P, et al. MRE11 mutations and impaired ATM-dependent responses in an Italian family with ataxia-telangiectasia-like disorder. Human Molecular Genetics. 2004;**13**(18):2155-2163

[26] Fernet M, Gribaa M, Salih MA, Seidahmed MZ, Hall J, Koenig M. Identification and functional consequences of a novel MRE11 mutation affecting 10 Saudi Arabian patients with the ataxia telangiectasia-like disorder. Human Molecular Genetics. 2005;**14**(2):307-318

[27] Aicardi J, Barbosa C, Andermann E, Andermann F, Morcos R, Ghanem Q, et al. Ataxia-ocular motor apraxia: a syndrome mimicking ataxia-telangiectasia. Annals of Neurology. 1988;**24**(4):497-502

[28] Le Ber I, Moreira MC, Rivaud-Péchoux S, Chamayou C, Ochsner F, Kuntzer T, et al. Cerebellar ataxia with oculomotor apraxia type 1: Clinical and genetic studies. Brain. 2003;**126**(Pt 12):2761-2772

[29] Le Ber I, Bouslam N, Rivaud-Péchoux S, Guimarães J, Benomar A, Chamayou C, et al. Frequency and phenotypic spectrum of ataxia with oculomotor apraxia 2: A clinical and genetic study in 18 patients. Brain. 2004;**127**(Pt 4):759-767

[30] Németh AH, Bochukova E, Dunne E, Huson SM, Elston J, Hannan MA, et al. Autosomal recessive cerebellar ataxia with oculomotor apraxia (ataxia-telangiectasia-like syndrome) is linked to chromosome 9q34. American Journal of Human Genetics. 2000;**67**(5):1320-1326

[31] Izatt L, Németh AH, Meesaq A, Mills KR, Taylor AM, Shaw CE. Autosomal recessive spinocerebellar ataxia and peripheral neuropathy with raised alpha-fetoprotein. Journal of Neurology. 2004;**251**(7):805-812

[32] Moreira MC, Klur S, Watanabe M, Németh AH, Le Ber I, Moniz JC, et al. Senataxin, the ortholog of a yeast RNA helicase, is mutant in ataxia-ocular apraxia 2. Nature Genetics. 2004;**36**(3):225-227

[33] Boder E. Ataxia-telangiectasia: An overview. Kroc Foundation Series. 1985;**19**:1-63

[34] Hoche F, Seidel K, Theis M, Vlaho S, Schubert R, Zielen S, et al. Neurodegeneration in ataxia telangiectasia: What is new? What is evident? Neuropediatrics. 2012;**43**(3):119-129

[35] Crawford TO. Ataxia telangiectasia. Seminars in Pediatric Neurology. 1998;**5**(4):287-294

[36] Boder E, Sedgwick RP. Ataxia-telangiectasia. (clinical and immunological aspects). Psychiatrie, Neurologie und Medizinische Psychologie. Beihefte. 1970;**13-14**:8-16

[37] Shaikh AG, Zee DS, Mandir AS, Lederman HM, Crawford TO. Disorders of upper limb movements in ataxia-telangiectasia. PLoS One. 2013;**8**(6):e67042

[38] Pearson TS. More than ataxia: Hyperkinetic movement disorders in childhood autosomal recessive ataxia syndromes. Tremor and Other Hyperkinetic Movements (N Y). 2016;**6**:368

[39] Sedgwick RP. Boder E. In: Vinken PJ, Bruyn GW, editors. Handbook of Clinical Neurology. Vol. 14. Amsterdam: North Holland Publishing; 1972

[40] Kwast O, Ignatowicz R. Progressive peripheral neuron degeneration in ataxia-telangiectasia: An electrophysiological study in children. Developmental Medicine and Child Neurology. 1990;**32**(9):800-807

[41] Sahama I, Sinclair K, Pannek K, Lavin M, Rose S. Radiological imaging in ataxia telangiectasia: a review. Cerebellum. 2014;**13**(4):521-530

[42] Kruman II, Wersto RP, Cardozo-Pelaez F, Smilenov L, Chan SL, Chrest FJ, et al. Cell cycle activation linked to neuronal cell death initiated by DNA damage. Neuron. 2004;**41**(4):549-561

[43] Lee Y, McKinnon PJ. Responding to DNA double strand breaks in the nervous system. Neuroscience. 2007;**145**(4):1365-1374

[44] Cabana MD, Crawford TO, Winkelstein JA, Christensen JR, Lederman HM. Consequences of the delayed diagnosis of ataxia-telangiectasia. Pediatrics. 1998;**102**(1 Pt 1):98-100

[45] Devaney R, Pasalodos S, Suri M, Bush A, Bhatt JM. Ataxia telangiectasia: presentation and diagnostic delay. Archives of Disease in Childhood. 2017;**102**(4):328-330

[46] Lin DD, Barker PB, Lederman HM, Crawford TO. Cerebral abnormalities in adults with ataxia-telangiectasia. AJNR.

American Journal of Neuroradiology. 2014;**35**(1):119-123

[47] Lewis RF, Lederman HM, Crawford TO. Ocular motor abnormalities in ataxia telangiectasia. Annals of Neurology. 1999;**46**(3):287-295

[48] Shaikh AG, Marti S, Tarnutzer AA, Palla A, Crawford TO, Straumann D, et al. Gaze fixation deficits and their implication in ataxia-telangiectasia. Journal of Neurology, Neurosurgery, and Psychiatry. 2009;**80**(8):858-864

[49] Shaikh AG, Marti S, Tarnutzer AA, Palla A, Crawford TO, Straumann D, et al. Ataxia telangiectasia: A "disease model" to understand the cerebellar control of vestibular reflexes. Journal of Neurophysiology. 2011;**105**(6):3034-3041

[50] Canny GJ, Roifman C, Weitzman S, Braudo M, Levison H. A pulmonary infiltrate in a child with ataxia telangiectasia. Annals of Allergy. 1988;**61**(6):422-3-466-8

[51] Nowak-Wegrzyn A, Crawford TO, Winkelstein JA, Carson KA, Lederman HM. Immunodeficiency and infections in ataxia-telangiectasia. The Journal of Pediatrics. 2004;**144**(4):505-511

[52] Lefton-Greif MA, Crawford TO, Winkelstein JA, Loughlin GM, Koerner CB, Zahurak M, et al. Oropharyngeal dysphagia and aspiration in patients with ataxia-telangiectasia. The Journal of Pediatrics. 2000;**136**(2):225-231

[53] Pagano G, Korkina LG, Brunk UT, Chessa L, Degan P, del Principe D, et al. Congenital disorders sharing oxidative stress and cancer proneness as phenotypic hallmarks: Prospects for joint research in pharmacology. Medical Hypotheses. 1998;**51**(3):253-266

[54] Umetsu DT, Ambrosino DM, Quinti I, Siber GR, Geha RS. Recurrent sinopulmonary infection and impaired antibody response to bacterial capsular polysaccharide antigen in children with selective IgG-subclass deficiency. The New England Journal of Medicine. 1985;**313**(20):1247-1251

[55] van Os NJH, Jansen AFM, van Deuren M, Haraldsson A, van Driel NTM, Etzioni A, et al. Ataxia-telangiectasia: Immunodeficiency and survival. Clinical Immunology. 2017;**178**:45-55

[56] McGrath-Morrow SA, Gower WA, Rothblum-Oviatt C, Brody AS, Langston C, Fan LL, et al. Evaluation and management of pulmonary disease in ataxia-telangiectasia. Pediatric Pulmonology. 2010;**45**(9):847-859

[57] McGrath-Morrow SA, Rothblum-Oviatt CC, Wright J, Schlechter H, Lefton-Greif MA, Natale VA, et al. Multidisciplinary Management of Ataxia Telangiectasia: Current perspectives. Journal of Multidisciplinary Healthcare. 2021;**14**:1637-1644

[58] McKinnon PJ. ATM and ataxia telangiectasia. EMBO Reports. 2004;**5**(8):772-776

[59] Stanley SE, Rao AD, Gable DL, McGrath-Morrow S, Armanios M. Radiation sensitivity and radiation necrosis in the short telomere syndromes. International Journal of Radiation Oncology, Biology, Physics. 2015;**93**(5):1115-1117

[60] Chen RL, Wang PJ, Hsu YH, Chang PY, Fang JS. Severe lung fibrosis after chemotherapy in a child with ataxia-telangiectasia. Journal of Pediatric Hematology/Oncology. 2002;**24**(1):77-79

[61] Schroeder SA, Swift M, Sandoval C, Langston C. Interstitial

lung disease in patients with ataxia-telangiectasia. Pediatric Pulmonology. 2005;**39**(6):537-543

[62] Bhatt JM, Bush A, van Gerven M, Nissenkorn A, Renke M, Yarlett L, et al. ERS statement on the multidisciplinary respiratory management of ataxia telangiectasia. European Respiratory Society. 2015;**24**(138):565-581

[63] Yalçin B, Kutluk MT, Sanal O, Akyüz C, Anadol D, Cağlar M, et al. Hodgkin's disease and ataxia telangiectasia with pulmonary cavities. Pediatric Pulmonology. 2002;**33**(5):399-403

[64] McGrath-Morrow SA, Lederman HM, Aherrera AD, Lefton-Greif MA, Crawford TO, Ryan T, et al. Pulmonary function in children and young adults with ataxia telangiectasia. Pediatric Pulmonology. 2014;**49**(1):84-90

[65] Brody AS. Thoracic CT technique in children. Journal of Thoracic Imaging. 2001;**16**(4):259-268

[66] Brenner DJ, Hall EJ. Computed tomography--an increasing source of radiation exposure. The New England Journal of Medicine. 2007;**357**(22):2277-2284

[67] Jeggo P. The role of the DNA damage response mechanisms after low-dose radiation exposure and a consideration of potentially sensitive individuals. Radiation Research. 2010;**174**(6):825-832

[68] Eibel R, Herzog P, Dietrich O, Rieger CT, Ostermann H, Reiser MF, et al. Pulmonary abnormalities in immunocompromised patients: Comparative detection with parallel acquisition MR imaging and thin-section helical CT. Radiology. 2006;**241**(3):880-891

[69] Montella S, Santamaria F, Salvatore M, Pignata C, Maglione M, Iacotucci P, et al. Assessment of chest high-field magnetic resonance imaging in children and young adults with noncystic fibrosis chronic lung disease: Comparison to high-resolution computed tomography and correlation with pulmonary function. Investigative Radiology. 2009;**44**(9):532-538

[70] Serra G, Milito C, Mitrevski M, Granata G, Martini H, Pesce AM, et al. Lung MRI as a possible alternative to CT scan for patients with primary immune deficiencies and increased radiosensitivity. Chest. 2011;**140**(6):1581-1589

[71] Driessen GJ, Ijspeert H, Weemaes CM, Haraldsson Á, Trip M, Warris A, et al. Antibody deficiency in patients with ataxia telangiectasia is caused by disturbed B- and T-cell homeostasis and reduced immune repertoire diversity. The Journal of Allergy and Clinical Immunology. 2013;**131**(5):1367-1375

[72] Sanal O, Ersoy F, Yel L, Tezcan I, Metin A, Ozyürek H, et al. Impaired IgG antibody production to pneumococcal polysaccharides in patients with ataxia-telangiectasia. Journal of Clinical Immunology. 1999;**19**(5):326-334

[73] Suarez F, Mahlaoui N, Canioni D, Andriamanga C, Dubois d'Enghien C, Brousse N, et al. Incidence, presentation, and prognosis of malignancies in ataxia-telangiectasia: A report from the French national registry of primary immune deficiencies. Journal of Clinical Oncology. 2015;**33**(2):202-208

[74] Noordzij JG, Wulffraat NM, Haraldsson A, Meyts I, van't Veer LJ, Hogervorst FB, et al. Ataxia-telangiectasia patients presenting with hyper-IgM syndrome.

Archives of Disease in Childhood. 2009;**94**(6):448-449

[75] Pietrucha BM, Heropolitańska-Pliszka E, Wakulińska A, Skopczyńska H, Gatti RA, Bernatowska E. Ataxia-telangiectasia with hyper-IgM and Wilms tumor: Fatal reaction to irradiation. Journal of Pediatric Hematology/Oncology. 2010;**32**(1):e28-e30

[76] Fiorilli M, Businco L, Pandolfi F, Paganelli R, Russo G, Aiuti F. Heterogeneity of immunological abnormalities in ataxia-telangiectasia. Journal of Clinical Immunology. 1983;**3**(2):135-141

[77] Cirillo E, Polizzi A, Soresina A, Prencipe R, Giardino G, Cancrini C, et al. Progressive depletion of B and T lymphocytes in patients with ataxia telangiectasia: Results of the Italian primary immunodeficiency network. Journal of Clinical Immunology. 2022;**42**(4):783-797

[78] McGrath-Morrow SA, Collaco JM, Detrick B, Lederman HM. Serum Interleukin-6 levels and pulmonary function in ataxia-telangiectasia. The Journal of Pediatrics. 2016;**171**:256-61.e1. DOI: 10.1016/j.jpeds.2016.01.002 Epub 2016 Feb 2

[79] McGrath-Morrow SA, Ndeh R, Collaco JM, Rothblum-Oviatt C, Wright J, O'Reilly MA, et al. Inflammation and transcriptional responses of peripheral blood mononuclear cells in classic ataxia telangiectasia. PLoS One. 2018;**13**(12):e0209496. DOI: 10.1371/journal.pone.0209496 eCollection 2018

[80] Patiroglu T, Gungor HE, Unal E, Kurtoglu S, Yikilmaz A, Patiroglu T. Hashimoto thyroiditis associated with ataxia telangiectasia. Journal of Pediatric Endocrinology & Metabolism. 2012;**25**(3-4):349-352

[81] Heath J, Goldman FD. Idiopathic thrombocytopenic purpura in a boy with ataxia telangiectasia on immunoglobulin replacement therapy. Journal of Pediatric Hematology/Oncology. 2010;**32**(1):e25-e27

[82] Alyasin S, Khoshkhui M, Abolnezhadian F. Autoimmune hemolytic anemia in a patient with probable ataxia telangiectasia: A case report. Iranian Journal of Immunology. 2014;**11**(3):217-220

[83] Chopra C, Davies G, Taylor M, Anderson M, Bainbridge S, Tighe P, et al. Immune deficiency in ataxia-telangiectasia: A longitudinal study of 44 patients. Clinical and Experimental Immunology. 2014;**176**(2):275-282

[84] Rothblum-Oviatt C, Wright J, Lefton-Greif MA, McGrath-Morrow SA, Crawford TO, Lederman HM. Ataxia telangiectasia: a review. Orphanet Journal of Rare Diseases. 2016;**11**(1):159

[85] Taylor AMR, Rothblum-Oviatt C, Ellis NA, Hickson ID, Meyer S, Crawford TO, et al. Chromosome instability syndromes. Nature Reviews. Disease Primers. 2019;**5**(1):64

[86] Stray-Pedersen A, Aaberge IS, Früh A, Abrahamsen TG. Pneumococcal conjugate vaccine followed by pneumococcal polysaccharide vaccine; immunogenicity in patients with ataxia-telangiectasia. Clinical and Experimental Immunology. 2005;**140**(3):507-516

[87] Chiam LY, Verhagen MM, Haraldsson A, Wulffraat N, Driessen GJ, Netea MG, et al. Cutaneous granulomas in ataxia telangiectasia and other primary immunodeficiencies: Reflection of inappropriate immune regulation? Dermatology. 2011;**223**(1):13-19

[88] Shoimer I, Wright N, Haber RM. Noninfectious granulomas: A sign of an

underlying immunodeficiency? Journal of Cutaneous Medicine and Surgery. 2016;**20**(3):259-262

[89] Bodemer C, Sauvage V, Mahlaoui N, Cheval J, Couderc T, Leclerc-Mercier S, et al. Live rubella virus vaccine long-term persistence as an antigenic trigger of cutaneous granulomas in patients with primary immunodeficiency. Clinical Microbiology and Infection. 2014;**20**(10):O656-O663

[90] Neven B, Pérot P, Bruneau J, Pasquet M, Ramirez M, Diana JS, et al. Cutaneous and visceral chronic granulomatous disease triggered by a rubella virus vaccine strain in children with primary Immunodeficiencies. Clinical Infectious Diseases. 2017;**64**(1):83-86

[91] Perelygina L, Plotkin S, Russo P, Hautala T, Bonilla F, Ochs HD, et al. Rubella persistence in epidermal keratinocytes and granuloma M2 macrophages in patients with primary immunodeficiencies. The Journal of Allergy and Clinical Immunology. 2016;**138**(5):1436-1439

[92] Cohen LE, Tanner DJ, Schaefer HG, Levis WR. Common and uncommon cutaneous findings in patients with ataxia-telangiectasia. Journal of the American Academy of Dermatology. 1984;**10**(3):431-438

[93] Ivonye C, Jamched U, Anderson D, Adesunloye B. Uncommon skin lesion in a patient with ataxia-telangiectasia. International Journal of Dermatology. 2008;**47**(10):1051-1052

[94] Pesce K, Rothe MJ. The premature aging syndromes. Clinics in Dermatology. 1996;**14**(2):161-170

[95] Lehman H. Skin manifestations of primary immune deficiency. Clinical Reviews in Allergy and Immunology. 2014;**46**(2):112-119

[96] Privette ED, Ram G, Treat JR, Yan AC, Heimall JR. Healing of granulomatous skin changes in ataxia-telangiectasia after treatment with intravenous immunoglobulin and topical mometasone 0.1% ointment. Pediatric Dermatology. 2014;**31**(6):703-707

[97] Iwata Y, Yoshizaki A, Komura K, Shimizu K, Ogawa F, Hara T, et al. CD19, a response regulator of B lymphocytes, regulates wound healing through hyaluronan-induced TLR4 signaling. The American Journal of Pathology. 2009;**175**(2):649-660

[98] Browne R, Cliffe L, Ip W, Brown K, McDermott E. A case of wild-type rubella-associated cutaneous granuloma in ataxia telangiectasia. Pediatric Dermatology. 2022;**39**(4):619-621

[99] Buchbinder D, Hauck F, Albert MH, Rack A, Bakhtiar S, Shcherbina A, et al. Rubella virus-associated cutaneous granulomatous disease: A unique complication in immune-deficient patients, not limited to DNA repair disorders. Journal of Clinical Immunology. 2019;**39**(1):81-89

[100] Stewart E, Prayle AP, Tooke A, Pasalodos S, Suri M, Bush A, et al. Growth and nutrition in children with ataxia telangiectasia. Archives of Disease in Childhood. 2016;**101**(12):1137-1141

[101] Ross LJ, Capra S, Baguley B, Sinclair K, Munro K, Lewindon P, et al. Nutritional status of patients with ataxia-telangiectasia: A case for early and ongoing nutrition support and intervention. Journal of Paediatrics and Child Health. 2015;**51**(8):802-807

[102] Voss S, Pietzner J, Hoche F, Taylor AM, Last JI, Schubert R, et al.

Growth retardation and growth hormone deficiency in patients with ataxia telangiectasia. Growth Factors. 2014;**32**(3-4):123-129

[103] Ersoy F, Berkel AI, Sanal O, Oktay H. Twenty-year follow-up of 160 patients with ataxia-telangiectasia. The Turkish Journal of Pediatrics. 1991;**33**(4):205-215

[104] Schubert R, Reichenbach J, Zielen S. Growth factor deficiency in patients with ataxia telangiectasia. Clinical and Experimental Immunology. 2005;**140**(3):517-519

[105] Peterson RD, Cooper MD, Good RA. Lymphoid tissue abnormalities associated with ataxia-telangiectasia. The American Journal of Medicine. 1966;**41**(3):342-359

[106] McFarlin DE, Strober W, Waldmann TA. Ataxia-telangiectasia. Medicine (Baltimore). 1972;**51**(4):281-314

[107] Zadik Z, Levin S, Prager-Lewin R, Laron Z. Gonadal dysfunction in patients with ataxia telangiectasia. Acta Paediatrica Scandinavica. 1978;**67**(4):477-479

[108] Worth PF, Srinivasan V, Smith A, Last JI, Wootton LL, Biggs PM, et al. Very mild presentation in adult with classical cellular phenotype of ataxia telangiectasia. Movement Disorders. 2013;**28**(4):524-528

[109] Andrade IGA, Costa-Carvalho BT, da Silva R, Hix S, Kochi C, Suano-Souza FI, et al. Risk of atherosclerosis in patients with ataxia telangiectasia. Annals of Nutrition & Metabolism. 2015;**66**(4):196-201

[110] Donath H, Hess U, Kieslich M, Theis M, Ohlenschläger U, Schubert R, et al. Diabetes in patients with ataxia telangiectasia: A National Cohort Study. Frontiers in Pediatrics. 2020;**8**:317

[111] Viswanathan P, Sharma Y, Maisuradze L, Tchaikovskaya T, Gupta S. Ataxia telangiectasia mutated pathway disruption affects hepatic DNA and tissue damage in nonalcoholic fatty liver disease. Experimental and Molecular Pathology. 2020;**113**:104369

[112] Paulino TL, Rafael MN, Hix S, Shigueoka DC, Ajzen SA, Kochi C, et al. Is age a risk factor for liver disease and metabolic alterations in ataxia telangiectasia patients? Orphanet Journal of Rare Diseases. 2017;**12**(1):136

[113] Yang DQ, Halaby MJ, Li Y, Hibma JC, Burn P. Cytoplasmic ATM protein kinase: An emerging therapeutic target for diabetes, cancer and neuronal degeneration. Drug Discovery Today. 2011;**16**(7-8):332-338

[114] Ditch S, Paull TT. The ATM protein kinase and cellular redox signaling: Beyond the DNA damage response. Trends in Biochemical Sciences. 2012;**37**(1):15-22

[115] Reiman A, Srinivasan V, Barone G, Last JI, Wootton LL, Davies EG, et al. Lymphoid tumours and breast cancer in ataxia telangiectasia; substantial protective effect of residual ATM kinase activity against childhood tumours. British Journal of Cancer. 2011;**105**(4):586-591

[116] Taylor AM, Metcalfe JA, Thick J, Mak YF. Leukemia and lymphoma in ataxia telangiectasia. Blood. 1996;**87**(2):423-438

[117] Ben Arush MW. Treatment of lymphoid malignancies in patients with ataxia-telangiectasia. Medical and Pediatric Oncology. 1999;**32**(6):479-480

[118] Sandoval C, Swift M. Hodgkin disease in ataxia-telangiectasia patients with poor outcomes. Medical and Pediatric Oncology. 2003;**40**(3):162-166

[119] Swift M, Morrell D, Massey RB, Chase CL. Incidence of cancer in 161 families affected by ataxia-telangiectasia. The New England Journal of Medicine. 1991;**325**(26):1831-1836

[120] Kulinski JM, Leonardo SM, Mounce BC, Malherbe L, Gauld SB, Tarakanova VL. Ataxia telangiectasia mutated kinase controls chronic gammaherpesvirus infection. Journal of Virology. 2012;**86**(23):12826-12837

[121] Seidemann K, Henze G, Beck JD, Sauerbrey A, Kühl J, Mann G, et al. Non-Hodgkin's lymphoma in pediatric patients with chromosomal breakage syndromes (AT and NBS): Experience from the BFM trials. Annals of Oncology. 2000;**11**(Suppl 1):141-145

[122] Machida S, Tomizawa D, Tamaichi H, Okawa T, Endo A, Imai K, et al. Successful treatment of diffuse large B-cell lymphoma in a patient with ataxia telangiectasia using rituximab. Journal of Pediatric Hematology/Oncology. 2013;**35**(6):482-485

[123] Olsen JH, Hahnemann JM, Børresen-Dale AL, Brøndum-Nielsen K, Hammarström L, Kleinerman R, et al. Cancer in patients with ataxia-telangiectasia and in their relatives in the nordic countries. Journal of the National Cancer Institute. 2001;**93**(2):121-127

[124] Marabelli M, Cheng SC, Parmigiani G. Penetrance of ATM gene mutations in breast cancer: A meta-analysis of different measures of risk. Genetic Epidemiology. 2016;**40**(5):425-431

[125] Perlman S, Becker-Catania S, Gatti RA. Ataxia-telangiectasia: Diagnosis and treatment. Seminars in Pediatric Neurology. 2003;**10**(3):173-182

[126] Hall MJ, Forman AD, Pilarski R, Wiesner G, Giri VN. Gene panel testing for inherited cancer risk. Journal of the National Comprehensive Cancer Network. 2014;**12**(9):1339-1346

[127] Gatti R, Perlman S. 1999 Mar 19 [Updated 2016 Oct 27]. Ataxia-Telangiectasia. In: Adam MP, Mirzaa GM, Pagon RA, Wallace SE, Bean LJH, Gripp KW, Amemiya a, Editors. GeneReviews® [Internet]. Seattle (WA): University of Washington, Seattle; 1993-2023

[128] Ataxia-Telangiectasia in Children: Guidance on Diagnosis and Clinical Care. http://www.atsociety.org.uk/data/files/William/A-T_Clinical_Guidance_Document_Final.pdf [Accessed: April 16, 2023].

[129] Boder E, Sedgwick R. Ataxia Telangiectasia: A Review of 101 Cases, in Little Club Clinics in Developmental Medicine No. 8. London: Heinemann Books; 1963. pp. 110-118

[130] Woods CG, Taylor AM. Ataxia telangiectasia in the British Isles: The clinical and laboratory features of 70 affected individuals. The Quarterly Journal of Medicine. 1992;**82**(298):169-179

[131] Kieslich M, Hoche F, Reichenbach J, Weidauer S, Porto L, Vlaho S, et al. Extracerebellar MRI-lesions in ataxia telangiectasia go along with deficiency of the GH/IGF-1 axis, markedly reduced body weight, high ataxia scores and advanced age. Cerebellum. 2010;**9**(2):190-197

[132] Lefton-Greif MA, Perlman AL, He X, Lederman HM, Crawford TO. Assessment of impaired coordination

between respiration and deglutition in children and young adults with ataxia telangiectasia. Developmental Medicine and Child Neurology. 2016;**58**(10):1069-1075

[133] Sun X, Becker-Catania SG, Chun HH, Hwang MJ, Huo Y, Wang Z, et al. Early diagnosis of ataxia-telangiectasia using radiosensitivity testing. The Journal of Pediatrics. 2002;**140**(6):724-731

[134] Stray-Pedersen A, Borresen-Dale AL, Paus E, Lindman CR, Burgers T, Abrahamsen TG. Alpha fetoprotein is increasing with age in ataxia-telangiectasia. European Journal of Paediatric Neurology. 2007;**11**(6):375-380

[135] Taylor AM, Byrd PJ. Molecular pathology of ataxia telangiectasia. Journal of Clinical Pathology. 2005;**58**(10):1009-1015

[136] Bower M. Diagnostic yield of targeted next generation sequencing approach in a young population: High frequency of recessive ataxias and implementation of a next generation sequencing copy-number variation. In: 5th Ataxia Investigators Meeting (AIM 2014). Las Vegas, NV; 2014

[137] Hellani A, Laugé A, Ozand P, Jaroudi K, Coskun S. Pregnancy after preimplantation genetic diagnosis for ataxia telangiectasia. Molecular Human Reproduction. 2002;**8**(8):785-788

[138] Verlinsky Y, Rechitsky S, S harapova T, Laziuk K, Barsky I, Verlinsky O, et al. Preimplantation diagnosis for immunodeficiencies. Reproductive Biomedicine Online. 2007;**14**(2):214-223

[139] Borte S, von Döbeln U, Fasth A, Wang N, Janzi M, Winiarski J, et al. Neonatal screening for severe primary immunodeficiency diseases using high-throughput triplex real-time PCR. Blood. 2012;**119**(11):2552-2555

[140] Mallott J, Kwan A, Church J, Gonzalez-Espinosa D, Lorey F, Tang LF, et al. Newborn screening for SCID identifies patients with ataxia telangiectasia. Journal of Clinical Immunology. 2013;**33**(3):540-549

[141] Herskind A, Greisen G, Nielsen JB. Early identification and intervention in cerebral palsy. Developmental Medicine and Child Neurology. 2015;**57**(1):29-36

[142] Cook A, Giunti P. Friedreich's ataxia: Clinical features, pathogenesis and management. British Medical Bulletin. 2017;**124**(1):19-30

[143] Pietrucha B, Heropolitańska-Pliszka E, Geffers R, Enßen J, Wieland B, Bogdanova NV, et al. Clinical and biological manifestation of RNF168 deficiency in two polish siblings. Frontiers in Immunology. 2017;**8**:1683

[144] Nissenkorn A, Hassin-Baer S, Lerman SF, Levi YB, Tzadok M, Ben-Zeev B. Movement disorder in ataxia-telangiectasia: Treatment with amantadine sulfate. Journal of Child Neurology. 2013;**28**(2):155-160

[145] van Egmond ME, Elting JW, Kuiper A, Zutt R, Heineman KR, Brouwer OF, et al. Myoclonus in childhood-onset neurogenetic disorders: The importance of early identification and treatment. European Journal of Paediatric Neurology. 2015;**19**(6):726-729

[146] Broccoletti T, Del Giudice E, Cirillo E, Vigliano I, Giardino G, Ginocchio VM, et al. Efficacy of very-low-dose betamethasone on neurological symptoms in ataxia-telangiectasia.

European Journal of Neurology. 2011;**18**(4):564-570

[147] Chessa L, Leuzzi V, Plebani A, Soresina A, Micheli R, D'Agnano D, et al. Intra-erythrocyte infusion of dexamethasone reduces neurological symptoms in ataxia teleangiectasia patients: Results of a phase 2 trial. Orphanet Journal of Rare Diseases. 2014;**9**:5

[148] Leuzzi V, Micheli R, D'Agnano D, Molinaro A, Venturi T, Plebani A, et al. Positive effect of erythrocyte-delivered dexamethasone in ataxia-telangiectasia. Neurology Neuroimmunology & Neuroinflammation. 2015;**2**(3):e98

[149] Pommerening H, van Dullemen S, Kieslich M, Schubert R, Zielen S, Voss S. Body composition, muscle strength and hormonal status in patients with ataxia telangiectasia: A cohort study. Orphanet Journal of Rare Diseases. 2015;**10**:155

[150] Lefton-Greif MA, Crawford TO, McGrath-Morrow S, Carson KA, Lederman HM. Safety and caregiver satisfaction with gastrostomy in patients with ataxia telangiectasia. Orphanet Journal of Rare Diseases. 2011;**6**:23

[151] Mitra A, Gooi J, Darling J, Newton-Bishop JA. Infliximab in the treatment of a child with cutaneous granulomas associated with ataxia telangiectasia. Journal of the American Academy of Dermatology. 2011;**65**(3):676-677

[152] Woelke S, Valesky E, Bakhtiar S, Pommerening H, Pfeffermann LM, Schubert R, et al. Treatment of granulomas in patients with ataxia telangiectasia. Frontiers in Immunology. 2018;**9**:2000

[153] Bakhtiar S, Woelke S, Huenecke S, Kieslich M, Taylor AM, Schubert R, et al. Pre-emptive allogeneic hematopoietic stem cell transplantation in ataxia telangiectasia. Frontiers in Immunology. 2018;**9**:2495

[154] Lavin MF, Gueven N, Bottle S, Gatti RA. Current and potential therapeutic strategies for the treatment of ataxia-telangiectasia. British Medical Bulletin. 2007;**81-82**:129-147

[155] Sandlund JT, Hudson MM, Kennedy W, Onciu M, Kastan MB. Pilot study of modified LMB-based therapy for children with ataxia-telangiectasia and advanced stage high grade mature B-cell malignancies. Pediatric Blood & Cancer. 2014;**61**(2):360-362

[156] Slack J, Albert MH, Balashov D, Belohradsky BH, Bertaina A, Bleesing J, et al. Outcome of hematopoietic cell transplantation for DNA double-strand break repair disorders. The Journal of Allergy and Clinical Immunology. 2018;**141**(1):322-328.e10. DOI: 10.1016/j.jaci.2017.02.036 Epub 2017 Apr 7

[157] Beier R, Sykora KW, Woessmann W, Maecker-Kolhoff B, Sauer M, Kreipe HH, et al. Allogeneic-matched sibling stem cell transplantation in a 13-year-old boy with ataxia telangiectasia and EBV-positive non-Hodgkin lymphoma. Bone Marrow Transplantation. 2016;**51**(9):1271-1274

[158] Ussowicz M, Musiał J, Duszeńko E, Haus O, Kałwak K. Long-term survival after allogeneic-matched sibling PBSC transplantation with conditioning consisting of low-dose busilvex and fludarabine in a 3-year-old boy with ataxia-telangiectasia syndrome and ALL. Bone Marrow Transplantation. 2013;**48**(5):740-741

[159] The Global A-T Family Data Platform. Available from: https://www.atfamilies.org/. [Accessed: April 16, 2023].

[160] Du L, Pollard JM, Gatti RA. Correction of prototypic ATM splicing mutations and aberrant ATM function with antisense morpholino oligonucleotides. Proceedings of the National Academy of Sciences of the United States of America. 2007;**104**(14):6007-6012

[161] Du L, Jung ME, Damoiseaux R, Completo G, Fike F, Ku JM, et al. A new series of small molecular weight compounds induce read through of all three types of nonsense mutations in the ATM gene. Molecular Therapy. 2013;**21**(9):1653-1660

Chapter 3

Childhood-Onset Ataxia

Daniela Munoz Chesta and Mónica Troncoso-Schifferli

Abstract

Childhood presentations of ataxia can often be challenging to diagnose. Recognising ataxia is especially difficult in young children, the most frequent reason for consultation is walking instability and loss of balance. Clinical presentations tend to be heterogeneous; key considerations may vary based on the age of onset, time course, and associated manifestations. Ataxias can be acute, intermittent, chronic non-progressive, or chronic progressive conditions. Acute ataxias are mostly acquired conditions (post-infectious or immune-mediated). Intermittent ataxias may be secondary to genetic channelopathies or metabolic diseases. Non-progressive chronic ataxias are mostly related to cerebellar malformations and progressive chronic ataxias are usually secondary to genetic variants, which in children are usually autosomal recessive conditions. A complete medical history and a detailed physical examination are essential for an adequate approach. Treatment of a child with ataxia depends on the aetiology. One of the most important challenges is to identify the treatable causes.

Keywords: gait, ataxia, cerebellar ataxia, paediatrics, childhood

1. Introduction

Diagnosing ataxia in the paediatric age is a challenge since children having difficulty in explaining the symptoms and their temporality and the differential diagnosis can be confusing. Children with ataxia classically present with a difficulty to ambulate often described as a "wide-based gait" [1]. Ataxia is especially incapacitating for children because they are still developing and learning motor abilities [2].

The prevalence of children's ataxia is not widely studied. More reports are focused on single conditions or include adults and paediatric patients. Musselman et al. have estimated the prevalence of ataxia in children is 26/100.000 children [3].

Recognising ataxia is especially difficult in young children, the most frequent reason for consultation is walking instability and loss of balance. History and physical examination represent the basis of the clinical approach [4, 5]. Initially, it is important to determine the temporality of the clinical symptom and elucidate the possible differential diagnosis. Past medical history, including birth history, development, medication, as well a complete family history should be obtained. A history of trauma, medication or toxic ingestion or, recent virus infection should be elicited especially in patients with acute ataxias [5]. In the cases of chronic ataxia, it is important to determine the presence of other neurological symptoms like seizures, sensory abnormalities, or movement disorders.

Physical examination should include skin inspection, looking for telangiectasias, xanthomas or ichthyosis. Neurological assessment must consider the evaluation of the child in a sitting position and during walking. It is important to elucidate if the ataxia is secondary to a cerebellum condition (cerebellar ataxia) or due to other areas of the nervous system (sensory ataxia, vestibular ataxia, etc.) [6]. Abnormal eye movements (abnormalities of saccadic eye movements, nystagmus), dysarthria, dysmetria and dysdiadochokinesis suggest cerebellar ataxia. Paresthesia, impaired position and vibration sense and positive Romberg sign suggest sensory ataxia).

The presence of other neurological signs such as speech disturbances, cognitive impairment, deep tendon reflex abnormalities, or the presence of chorea, dystonia, or myoclonus may be clues to the diagnosis.

Ataxia in children can be in different ways, depending on neuroanatomy (sensory or cerebellar aetiology (primary or secondary), and temporal course [7]. Temporally, ataxia can be divided into two other groups: acute and chronic. Acute ataxias are usually secondary ataxias, whereas chronic ataxia may be either primary or secondary. Chronic ataxias are divided into intermitted or persistent ataxias. Persistent ataxias are divided into progressive and non progressive conditions [6].

2. Acute ataxias

Acutely presenting ataxia is a relatively common presentation to paediatric acute services or child neurologists though the cause of acute ataxia is most often benign, it is important during initial evaluation to recognise or exclude serious causes including brain tumour and central nervous system infections [8]. The most common causes are intoxication and acute cerebellar ataxia (ACA) (**Table 1**).

Causes of Acute Ataxias
Intoxications (alcohol, drugs)
Stroke
Trauma
Brain tumour
Brainstem encephalitis
Opsoclonus Mioclonus
Miller Fisher variant of Guillain Barre Syndrome
Multiple Sclerosis
ADEM
Acute cerebellitis
Labyrinthitis
Basilar migraine
Benign paroxysmal vertigo

Table 1.
Causes of acute ataxia.

2.1 Intoxications

Ingestion of a toxin represents approximately 30% of acute children ataxia cases [9]. The accidental ingestion of prescription and nonprescription medications is more frequent in children less than 6 years of age [9]. Benzodiazepines are the most common drug reported, nevertheless other medications such as carbamazepine, phenytoin, phenobarbital, lamotrigine, dextromethorphan (main ingredient of cough suppressant) [10, 11] and antineoplastic or immunosuppressive drugs such as cyclosporine, tacrolimus may cause ataxia [12]. Toxic agents that may be related to ataxia include lithium, ethanol and marijuana [6, 13].

Toxin ingestion may manifest with ataxia associated with mental status changes such as lethargy, confusion, inappropriate speech, or impaired consciousness level. Toxicology screening tests are commonly performed in the initial evaluation of acute ataxia in children [14].

2.2 Acute cerebellar ataxia

Acute cerebellar ataxia is the most common cause of acute ataxia in children accounting for nearly 30–50% of all cases [9]. It is a benign and self-limiting syndrome, usually a postinfectious phenomenon. It usually occurs in children between the ages of 3 and 5, but it can be seen in older children [9, 15]. The main clinical manifestation is sudden onset of unsteadiness of gait associated with cerebellar signs, nystagmus is reported in nearly 50% of patients [15]. Ataxia usually starts 1–3 weeks following a viral infection. Different viral agents have been linked to its development; the most common virus associated is varicella (25%) and it can occur in association with vaccines [12]. It has a benign prognosis with spontaneous recovery in most cases, the average duration of cerebellar signs is about 8 weeks [15].

2.3 Postinfectious cerebellitis

Postinfectious cerebellitis is a manifestation of one severe end of a continuous clinical spectrum, with acute cerebellar ataxia representing the milder end. Patients with postinfectious cerebellitis have ataxia and other symptoms, such as vomiting, abnormal mental status, or seizures. It is associated with abnormal brain imaging results due to cerebellar oedema]. Unlike acute cerebellar ataxia, the outcomes of postinfectious cerebellitis are not always favourable and may need aggressive management.

2.4 Acute disseminated encephalomyelitis

ADEM is an acute immune-mediated demyelinating encephalopathy with or without myelitis that is usually preceded by a viral infection. ADEM may present with prodromal signs such as fever, vomiting, or headache. Ataxia is a common feature (42%). Other neurological manifestations include long pathway signs (71%), acute hemiparesis (64%), consciousness impairment (58%), cranial nerve palsies (37%), meningeal reaction (36%), seizures (29%), visual loss due to optic neuritis (19%) and spinal cord involvement (20%) [16]. Diagnosis requires the demonstration of characteristic multifocal demyelinating lesions on MRI (**Figure 1**). The approximate incidence of ADEM is 0.2–0.4 per 100,000 children annually [16, 17]. The most common age of presentation is 3 to 7 years [18].

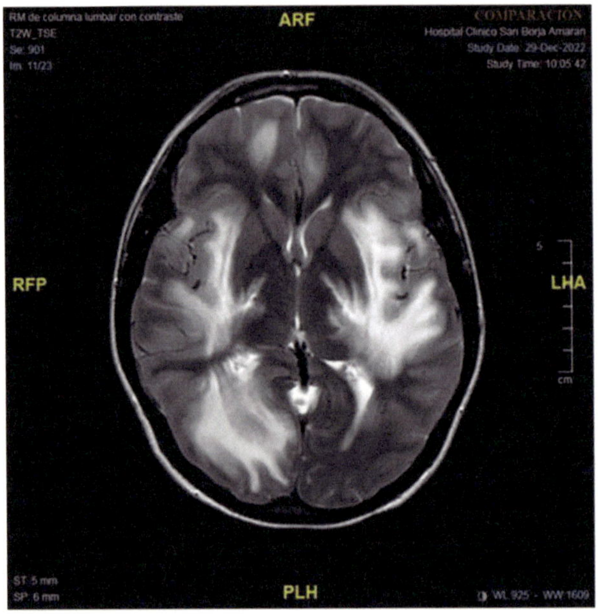

Figure 1.
Multifocal demyelinating lesions on MRI T2 weighted imaging sequence in a patient with ADEM.

Current first-line therapy is methylprednisolone at 20–30 mg/kg IV once a day for 3–5 days, followed by a corticosteroid taper over 4–6 weeks [19]. ADEM typically has a monophasic evolution with a favourable prognosis with complete recovery in almost all the patients usually over 4–6 weeks [20]. There is evidence that a minority of children may have persistent and long-term effects, such as physical or cognitive deficits, including attention difficulties and poor executive functioning [21, 22].

2.5 Opsoclonus-myoclonus syndrome

Opsoclonus-myoclonus syndrome (OMS) is a rare autoimmune neurological disorder that can occur in both children and adults. In childhood OMS, the main age of onset is approximately 18 months [23, 24]. Classic manifestations include an acute or subacute onset of ataxia, opsoclonus and myoclonic jerks associated with irritability and sleep disturbance [25]. All the main features may not be present initially and the diagnosis may be delayed weeks or months from the onset of symptoms.

OMS can be idiopathic, parainfectious or occur as a paraneoplastic syndrome. The most frequent neoplasia associated with childhood OMS in neuroblastoma. Neuroblastoma is present in at least 50% of affected children, and OMS presents as a paraneoplastic syndrome in 2–3% of all children with neuroblastomas [26]. Children with neuroblastoma and OMS have a better prognosis for their oncologic disease since they are usually diagnosed at earlier tumour stages and neuroblastoma is better differentiated [25].

The management and outcome depend on the aetiology and the spread of the disease. A regular response of neurological symptoms to immunosuppressive treatment is described. However, although the main neurological symptoms may show a good response, most children remain severe neuropsychological alterations [23].

2.6 Central nervous system tumours

Central nervous system tumours are the most frequent neoplasia among those aged 0–19 years with an incidence rate of 6.14 per 100,000 population, representing the second cause of death from cancer in childhood [27]. Posterior fossa tumours account for 45–60% of all paediatric brain tumours [28]. Most posterior brain tumours are discovered between 3 and 11 years old [27].

Ataxia associated with posterior fossa brain tumours, in the absence of haemorrhage or acute CSF obstruction, tends to be subacute and is associated with symptoms of increased intracranial pressure (headache, vomiting). Treatment of brain tumours includes surgery, chemotherapy, radiotherapy, and rehabilitation. The prognosis is variable and depends on the type of tumour and localization (**Figure 2A** and **B**).

2.7 Anti: N-methyl-D-aspartate (NMDA) receptor encephalitis

Anti–Nmethyl-D-aspartate (NMDA) receptor encephalitis is a common, autoimmune cause of encephalitis in children. Clinical manifestations usually include abnormal behaviour, change in mental status, speech difficulties, seizures, movement disorders and autonomic dysfunction [29]. Cerebellar ataxia has been described as the initial symptom [30] and during the first months of the disease associated with the other clinical manifestations [31, 32].

2.8 Others

Other causes of acute ataxia in children are Guillain-Barré syndrome, Miller-Fisher syndrome, Bickerstaff brainstem encephalitis, transverse myelitis, stroke, venous sinus thrombosis, meningitis, rhombencephalitis, labyrinthitis, basilar migraine, benign paroxysmal vertigo, cerebellar abscess and celiac disease, among others [8, 33, 34].

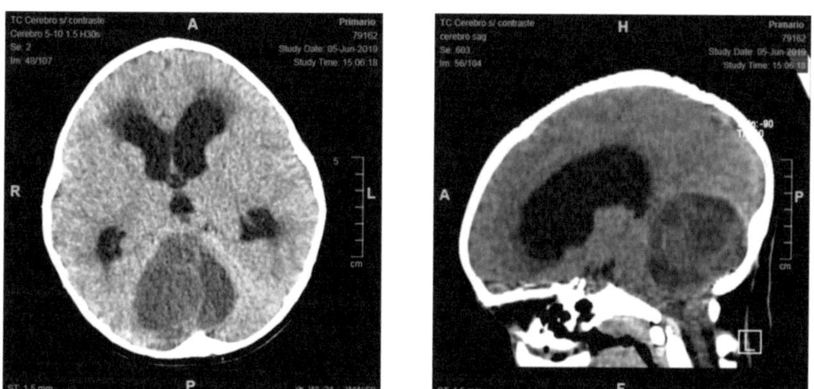

Figure 2.
Head CT scan examination (A) axial section and (B) sagittal section demonstrated an inhomogeneous hyperdense lesion in the posterior fossa.

3. Intermittent ataxias

Intermittent ataxias occur infrequently in paediatrics and are defined as ataxia that recurs after complete or almost complete resolution of an acute or subacute episode of ataxia [35]. The main causes of recurrent ataxia are genetic episodic ataxias; other causes are inflammatory and metabolic diseases (**Table 2**).

3.1 Episodic ataxias

Episodic ataxias (EAs) are a clinically and genetically heterogeneous group of autosomal dominant inherited channelopathies characterised by recurrent episodes of cerebellar ataxia [36]. EAs usually start during childhood or adolescence. Ataxia episodes can vary from seconds to hours or days and are often triggered by different specific stimuli [37]. Eight different forms of autosomal dominant or familial AD are currently identified [38]. EA1 and EA2, represent the most prevalent group of EAs patients and have recognisable ictal and interictal phenotypes [37].

EA1 is associated with mutations in a voltage-gated K channel gene (KCNA1) [36]. EA1 begins usually in childhood and ataxic episodes are associated with vertigo [38]. In EA1 the episodes are frequent, brief (seconds to minutes) and are triggered by abrupt exercise, stress, startle, fever, caffeine or alcohol [38, 39]. Dysarthria, tremors, diplopia, blurred vision, vertigo, nausea, migraine, or diaphoresis may also be present during the ataxia episodes. Between attacks, EA 1 is associated with myokymia [38]. Approximately 20% of EA1 individuals evolve with persistent cerebellar symptoms [37]. Different medications have been reported to be effective in EA1, including acetazolamide (AZT), carbamazepine and valproic acid [37, 38].

EA2 is caused by heterozygous variants in the calcium channel, voltage-dependent, P/Q type, and α1A subunit (CACNA1A) gene [38]. EA 2 usually presents with recurrent episodes of ataxia that last up to several hours or days and the frequency of the attacks ranges from four times per week to once per year [37]. During the attack, patients can

Causes of Intermittent Ataxias
Autosomal Dominant Episodic Ataxias
Basilar Migraine
Benign paroxysmal vertigo
Multiple Sclerosis
Metabolic Disorders
Urea cycle defects
• Aminoacidopathies (e.g., Maple syrup disease)
• Pyruvate dehydrogenase deficiency
• Pyruvate decarboxylase deficiency
• Glut 1 deficiency
• CAPOS syndrome
Relapsing opsoclonus-myoclonus syndrome

Table 2.
Causes of intermittent ataxia.

also manifest Vertigo and dizziness, dysarthria, migraine, nausea and vomiting, diplopia, tinnitus, and generalised muscle weakness. Ataxic episodes are triggered by emotional stress, exercise, phenytoin, and caffeine but not by startle [36]. Clinical onset is usually in the first two decades of life, although late-onset cases have been reported [38]. In EA2 often an interictal downbeat nystagmus with other cerebellar dysfunctions is present [38]. Acetazolamide is the first line treatment for EA2, patients unresponsive to or unable to tolerate acetazolamide may respond to 4-aminopyridine [39].

3.2 Glucose transporter type 1 deficiency

Glucose transporter type 1 (Glut1) deficiency syndrome is caused by heterozygous, mostly de novo, mutations in the SLC2A1 gene encoding the glucose transporter GLUT1. This glucose transporter is the most important energy carrier of the brain through the blood–brain barrier [40]. Glut1 deficiency syndrome is classically characterised by the presence of childhood epilepsy, developmental delay, acquired microcephaly, cognitive impairment, spasticity, ataxia, and dystonia.

Paroxysmal manifestations including seizures and nonepileptic paroxysmal episodes are also part of the phenotype [40, 41]. Clinical severity may vary from mild to severe neurological dysfunction. In children with mild phenotypes, paroxysmal manifestations, such as exercise-induced dyskinesia or episodic ataxia, may be the only manifestations of this condition [41]. Low CSF level of glucose is a characteristic finding in Glut1 deficiency syndrome and mutation analysis of the SLC2A1 gene confirms the diagnosis [38].

The ketogenic diet provides an alternative source of energy by switching brain metabolism from glucose to ketone bodies, it is considered the gold standard treatment and can improve or reverse symptoms, especially if started as early as possible.

3.3 CAPOS syndrome

CAPOS syndrome, named after its symptoms (cerebellar ataxia, areflexia, pes cavus, optic atrophy, and sensorineural hearing loss) is a rare condition caused by variants in the ATP1A3 gene that encodes the α3 subunit of Na^{+}/K^{+} -ATPase, an integral membrane protein responsible for the regulation of sodium and potassium concentrations over the cell membrane [42]. Three classic phenotypes (rapid-onset parkinsonian dystonia, alternating infantile hemiplegia, and CAPOS syndrome) were initially described, but recently an increasing number of cases presenting with atypical and overlapping features have been reported [43].

The symptoms usually start in childhood between 1 and 5 years of age, and patients typically present an acute episode of fever-induced ataxia associated with encephalopathic features and weakness [42, 43]. Recovery from the episode is complete in most cases and a recurrent course is characteristic. Afterwards, the patients show a slow progression of the disease [42, 44]. Patients classically experience two to three episodes of acute ataxia during life before transitioning to a slowly progressive evolution [44]. There is no specific treatment for CAPOS syndrome, acetazolamide has been used to prevent relapses of the acute episodes [42].

3.4 Others

Other causes of intermittent ataxia in children include metabolic disorders like pyruvate dehydrogenase deficiency [45, 46], pyruvate decarboxylase deficiency, urea cycle defects, aminoacidopathies, organic acidopathies, recurrent ADEM, multiple sclerosis, benign paroxysmal vertigo [36], vestibular migraine, between others [35].

4. Chronic non-progressive ataxias

Chronic non-progressive ataxias are conditions that manifest with chronic ataxia with a stable (non-progressive) evolution. In this group are included congenital ataxias and their four subgroups recently proposed: cerebellar malformation, syndromic congenital ataxias, congenital cerebellar hypoplasia, and pontocerebellar hypoplasia [47]. Cerebellar structural disruption related to congenital infectious, tumours and stroke are also chronic non-progressive ataxias (**Table 3**).

4.1 Congenital ataxia

Congenital ataxias (CA) are a genetically heterogeneous group of disorders characterised by the presence of varying degrees of motor and language developmental delay, very early-onset cerebellar ataxia, cognitive impairment, and hypotonia [48]. Other common features include seizures, ocular signs (nystagmus, strabismus), behaviour changes, and microcephaly. Most cases have a non-progressive course, and patients report improvement in their motor and cognitive skills over time [47]. Recently, Raslan et al. [47] have proposed to classify CA into four categories:

- Cerebellar Malformations: patients with structural changes of the cerebellum. Neuroimaging is mandatory for the diagnosis. Cerebellar Malformations include Dandy-Walker malformation (hypoplasia of the cerebellar vermis, cystic dilation of the fourth ventricle, and an enlarged posterior fossa with upward displacement of the lateral sinuses, tentorium, and torcular) [49], rombencephalosynapsis, macrocerebellum, pontine tegmental cap dysplasia and cerebella dysplasia.

- Syndromic Congenital Ataxias: a group of conditions that associate specific dysmorphic characteristics, cerebellar hypoplasia, and early ataxia as the main feature. Syndromic congenital ataxias include Joubert Syndrome (characterised clinically by hypotonia progressing to ataxia, global developmental delay, ocular motor apraxia, and breathing dysregulation associated with the presence of the molar tooth sign on brain imaging consisting of elongated and thickened of the superior cerebellar peduncles) [50], Gillespie syndrome (iris hypoplasia, cognitive impairment and

Causes of Chronic Non-Progressive Ataxias
Congenital Ataxia (CA)
• Cerebellar Malformations
• Syndromic Congenital Ataxias (e.g., Joubert Syndrome)
• Congenital Cerebellar Hypoplasia
• Pontocerebellar Hypoplasia
Cerebellar structural disruption secondary to congenital infectious, tumours and stroke

Table 3.
Causes of chronic non-progressive ataxias.

cerebella hypoplasia), Dekaban-Arima syndrome (agenesis or hypoplasia of vermis, congenital polycystic kidneys, and hepatic disease), among others [47].

- Congenital Cerebellar Hypoplasia: In children with cerebellar hypoplasia as a main feature in neuroimaging, ataxia is frequently associated with cognitive impairment. Some genes have been linked with specific phenotypes and structural disorders of the cerebellum, including CACNA1A, CAMTA1, TUBA1A, TUBA8, RELN, OPHN1 genes [47].

- Pontocerebellar Hypoplasia: a group of heterogeneous conditions characterised by cerebellar and brainstem hypoplasia. Clinical manifestations include severe global development delay associated with dysmorphic features, microcephaly, optic atrophy, spasticity, epilepsy, and movement disorders [51]. Thirteen different types are described (from PCH1 to PCH 13) [47].

5. Chronic progressive ataxias

Chronic progressive ataxias are usually inherited ataxias that include a heterogeneous group of clinically and genetically distinguished neurodegenerative disorders. Depending on its inherence chronic ataxias are classified in autosomal dominant, autosomal recessive, and X-linked ataxias (**Table 4**).

Principal Causes of Chronic Progressive Ataxias
Primary Autosomal Recessive Ataxias
Friedreich Ataxia
Ataxia Telangiectasia
Ataxia with vitamin E deficiency
Ataxia with oculomotor apraxia 1 and 2
Ataxia with coenzyme Q deficiency
Abetalipoproteinemia
Cerebrotendinous xanthomatosis
Autosomal recessive ataxia of Charlevoix-Saguenay (ARSACS)
Other metabolic or complex autosomal recessive disorders that have ataxia as an associated feature
Niemann Pick C
Refsum Disease
Vanishing white matter disease
Wilson disease
Biotinidase Deficiency
Lafora Disease
Tay-Sachs disease
Sandhoff disease
Glut 1 deficiency
Hartnup disease
GM1 gangliosidosis type II

Table 4.
Causes of chronic progressive ataxias.

5.1 Autosomal dominant ataxias

Autosomal dominant ataxias usually presenting as spinocerebellar ataxia (SCAs). SCAs are rare in children and the clinical clue for the diagnosis is the identification of family history [7]. Most common SCAs are caused by an expansion of a CAG trinucleotide repeat in the respective gene, therefore an anticipation phenomenon can occur in some families.

Infantile and childhood onset has been described in SCA2, SCA7, SCA10, SCA13, SCA14, SCA21, SCA25, SCA28, SCA42, SCA44, and DRPLA (dentatorubral-pallido-luysian atrophy) [52].

5.2 Autosomal recessive ataxias

Autosomal recessive ataxias are a group of complex genetic ataxia disorders associated with variable central and peripheral involvement and systemic manifestations. A new clinical and pathophysiological classification of autosomal recessive cerebellar ataxia has recently become available [53] and is a very useful tool for the initial clinical approach to a patient presenting with ataxia. There is a long list of disorders associated with autosomal recessive ataxias, some of which are described below.

Autosomal recessive ataxias are a group of complex genetic ataxia disorders associated with variable central and peripheral involvement and systemic manifestations. A new clinical and pathophysiological classification of autosomal recessive cerebellar ataxia has recently become available [53]. This classification separates autosomal recessive ataxias in two groups: primary autosomal recessive cerebellar ataxias and complex multisystem disorders that are associated with ataxia. There is a long list of disorders associated with autosomal recessive ataxias, some of which are described below.

5.3 Primary autosomal recessive cerebellar ataxias

5.3.1 Friedreich ataxia

Friedreich Ataxia (FA) is caused by mutations in the FXN gene (9q21.11), which encodes the synthesis of frataxin, a protein that is involved in mitochondrial function. Its deficiency leads to mitochondrial iron overload, defective energy supply and generation of reactive oxygen species. Most patients carry homozygous GAA expansions in the first intron of the frataxin gene on chromosome 9 [54].

FA age of onset has a wide range, which can go from 5 to 25 years of age, although cases of late-onset (after 25 years of age) and very late onset (after 40 years of age) have been described [55]. Usually, the onset of symptoms is between the ages of 10 and 16 with gait instability [54]. The classical phenotype of FA is associated with progressive sensory and cerebellar ataxia, with areflexia, loss of position or vibration sensation, pes cavus, Babinski sign, and scoliosis. Patients usually become wheelchair-bound after a mean disease duration of 10–15 years [56]. Other neurological manifestations include dysmetria, dysarthria, and auditory and optic neuropathy. FA patients also have systemic complications, including cardiomyopathy and diabetes [57]. MRI usually shows spinal atrophy [54]. Currently, there is no effective treatment to delay neurodegeneration in Friedreich's ataxia, but different newer treatments are now being studied.

5.3.2 Ataxia telangiectasia

Ataxia-telangiectasia (AT) is the second most common autosomal recessive hereditary ataxia in children [7]. AT is caused by a mutation in the AMT gene, which encodes a kinase protein involved in DNA repair [58]. The onset of symptoms is usually in early childhood, classical neurological signs include progressive cerebellar ataxia, oculomotor apraxia, chorea and cognitive dysfunction [59]. Scleral and cutaneous telangiectasias are characteristic of AT, although they may be absent initially. Other systemic manifestations include variable immunodeficiency with recurrent infections, radiosensitivity, susceptibility to malignancies, poor growth and insulin-resistant diabetes [60]. Serum elevation of carcinoembryonic antigen and alpha-fetoprotein are constant markers. Immunoglobulins are typically decreased and MRI classically shows marked atrophy of the cerebellum [61]. AT patients have a poor prognosis, and average life expectancy was reported to be approximately 25 years [60]. No curative therapy is available for ataxia-telangiectasia.

5.3.3 Ataxia with oculomotor apraxia type 1 (AOA1) and type 2 (AOA2)

Both recessive conditions manifest as the main clinical features of ataxia and oculomotor apraxia. AOA1 is caused by mutations in the APTX gene which encodes a nuclear protein called aprataxin that is involved in DNA repair [62]. Ataxia usually begins during the first decade of life and is often associated with neuropathy, chorea, nystagmus, and oculomotor apraxia [62]. AOA1 patients do not have extra neurological manifestations. Most AOA1 patients lose the ability to walk independently approximately 7–10 years after the first symptoms [7]. Hypoalbuminemia and hypercholesterolemia are frequent [63].

AOA2 is caused by mutations in the SETX gene which encodes the synthesis of senataxin, a helicase considered to be involved in the defence against DNA damage [64]. Usually, the onset of the disease occurs between 12 and 22 years of age (later than AOA1) [65]. The most frequent presenting manifestation is cerebellar ataxia, which is slowly progressive. Oculomotor apraxia may be absent. Other clinical manifestations include strabismus, sensorimotor peripheral neuropathy and different movement disorders (specially chorea and dystonia) [64, 65]. Elevated serum AFP levels are characteristic, and creatine kinase (CK) levels are occasionally elevated. Cerebellar atrophy appears to be an early sign of AOA2, which stabilises after several years after disease onset [64].

5.3.4 Ataxia with vitamin E deficiency

Ataxia with vitamin E deficiency (AVED) is caused by variants in the APTT gene, which encodes the synthesis of the alpha-tocopherol transfer protein, responsible for incorporating vitamin E into very low-density proteins in the liver, which will transport it to the brain. The first manifestations are observed between 4 and 18 years of age in individuals with or without a history of malabsorption disorders [66]. Subjects with AVED develop a neurological phenotype very similar to Friedreich's ataxia [67]. AVED is characterised by progressive ataxia, areflexia, head tremor, loss of proprioception and retinitis pigmentosa [68]. Supplementation improves symptoms and prevents the progression of the disease [68].

5.3.5 Autosomal-recessive spastic ataxia of Charlevoix: Saguenay

Autosomal-recessive spastics ataxia of Charlevoix Saguenay (ARSACS) is caused by mutations in the SACS gene which is located on chromosome 13q12.12 [69]. SACS gene encodes sacsin, a protein that has chaperone activity and interacts with the proteasome, but is also involved in mitochondrial function and affects axonal and dendritic transport [70]. The mean age at onset is approximately 6 years (range: 0–40 years) [71]. ARSACS is clinically characterised by early-onset progressive cerebellar ataxia, spasticity and peripheral neuropathy. Oculomotor disturbances and dysarthria are also common manifestations. A characteristic finding is the presence of yellow streaks of hypermyelinated fibres radiating from the edges of the optic disc seen on ophthalmologic examination. In the optical coherence tomography study, an increase in the thickness of the retinal fibre layer can be observed [72]. MRI imaging shows atrophy of the cerebellar vermis, atrophy of the posterior part of the corpus callosum, and linear hypointensities in the pons on T2 and T2-FLAIR [73].

5.4 Other metabolic or complex autosomal recessive disorders that have ataxia as an associated feature

5.4.1 Niemann-pick disease type C

Niemann-Pick disease (PC) is caused by autosomal recessive mutations in either the NPC1 or NPC2 gene. NP1 encodes a transmembrane protein and NP2 an intralysosomal protein, the deficiency of which results in the intracellular accumulation of cholesterol and complex lipids, such as sphingolipids and phospholipids, within the endosomal/lysosomal system [74]. NPC has a heterogeneous spectrum of signs and symptoms in visceral, neurologic, and psychiatric domains, with characteristic symptomatology depending on the age of onset. Ataxia is a frequent manifestation in late infantile, juvenile and adult forms and can be associated with vertical gaze palsy, epilepsy, dystonia and cataplexy [75]. The prognosis is correlated with the age at onset of the neurological manifestations, with early-onset forms progressing more rapidly than late-onset forms [74]. MRI and CT may be normal or show cerebellar or cortical atrophy [76].

5.4.2 Wilson disease (WD)

Wilson Disease (WD) is caused by mutations in the ATP7B gene, which encodes the synthesis of an ATPase that participates in the copper transport, located preferentially in the liver but also in the brain [77]. WD generally presents in childhood and young adulthood. The most common age of presentation is 10 to 20 years [78]. WD have different forms of presentation, including fulminant hepatitis, psychosis, or neurological disorder (tremor, dystonia, akinetic-rigid syndrome, and ataxia). A characteristic ophthalmological manifestation includes the Kayser-Fleischer ring [79]. MRI imaging findings are variable, with neurological patients classically presenting with bilateral high signal intensities on T2 and Flair-weighted images in the basal ganglia, the mesencephalon and the cerebellum [77]. Low levels of ceruloplasmin and copper are detected in the blood, the excretion of which is increased in urine [78]. D-penicillamine and trientine as chelators, and tetrathiomolybdate and zinc sulfate are the usual treatment [79].

5.4.3 Vanishing white matter disease

Vanishing White Matter Disease (VWM) is an autosomal recessive leukoencephalopathy, most often with onset in childhood. The classic phenotype is characterised by chronic progressive neurological deterioration, especially cerebellar ataxia, with additional episodes of rapid deterioration after minor head trauma and febrile infections possibly leading to coma or death [80]. MRI shows a diffuse cerebral white matter abnormality, beginning in the presymptomatic stage. Subsequently, the affected white matter disappears and is replaced by fluid (**Figure 3**) [80].

6. Ataxias scales in children

Ataxia scales are used especially in clinical trials evaluating the potential effect of therapeutic agents. Different ataxia rating scales have been used in the paediatric age, the most commonly applied in children include the International Cooperative Ataxia Rating Scale (ICARS) and the Scale for Ataxia Assessment and Rating (SARA) [81].

ICARS was initially developed to evaluate treatment efficacy in randomised clinical trials. ICARS is constituted by four clinical subscales domains including posture and gait, limb coordination, speech and oculomotor function [81]. ICARS ranges from 0 (optimal outcome) to 100 (most severely affected outcome). In children, some reports are suggesting an age-dependent ICARS score, with performance improving with age [82].

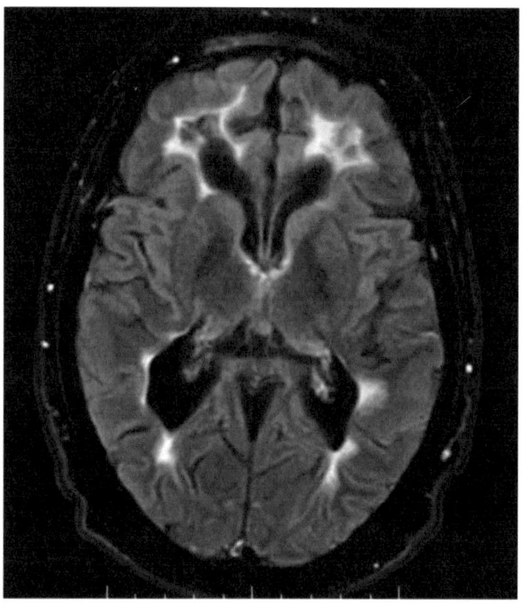

Figure 3.
MRI FLAIR sequence revealed diffuse white matter hyperintensity and interspersed areas of low signal intensities findings in classic vanishing white matter (VWM) disease.

SARA includes eight items that range a total score from 0 (no ataxia) to 40 (most severe ataxia), assessing gait, stance, sitting, speech disturbance, finger chase, nose-to-finger test, fast alternating hand movements, and heel-shin slide. Studies also indicate an exponential decline of SARA scores [83] with age, and some authors do not recommend its use in children under 12 years of age [84].

In both mentioned scales, the presence of different types of movement disorders can influence scores, so its application in uniform phenotypes of movement disorders is suggested for an adequate interpretation [85].

7. Treatment of childhood ataxias

Treatment of a child with ataxia depends on the aetiology. One of the most important challenges is to identify the treatable causes. For example, ataxia with vitamin E deficiency (AVED), abetalipoproteinemia, and hypobetalipoproteinemia are treated with vitamin E. Wilson's disease is treated with D-penicillamine and trientine as copper chelators. Some metabolic disorders are treated with dietary modifications, such as glutamate 1 deficiency and pyruvate dehydrogenase deficiency, which are treated with the ketogenic diet. Specific enzymatic treatments have recently been developed for some metabolic disorders, especially focused on slowing down their progression. An example is Miglustat for NPC patients [74].

Physical therapy is an important part of treatment to help maintain mobility as long as possible. Occupational therapy, and speech or language therapy are also part of the symptomatic therapy [86].

There are also reports of some benefits in adults with cerebellar ataxia with transcranial magnetic stimulation [87] and transcranial direct current stimulation [88], but the evidence is still lacking, especially in children.

8. Conclusions and final remarks

Ataxia can be difficult to diagnose in children. It may be undetected mainly in very young children and incorrectly related to a delay of coordination. The differential diagnosis of ataxia remains challenging. An increasing number of diseases are described, and the phenotypes are not always typical. A complete medical history and a detailed physical examination are keys to an adequate approach. It is important to always identify the time course of onset and associated manifestations. The causes of ataxia are various and have different prognoses that can range from transient and benign to particularly severe conditions. Ataxias manifest in various forms: acute, intermittent, chronic non-progressive, and chronic progressive. Acute ataxias predominantly arise from acquired causes such as post-infectious or immune-mediated conditions. Intermittent ataxias may stem from genetic channelopathies or metabolic disorders. Non-progressive chronic ataxias primarily result from cerebellar malformations, whereas progressive chronic ataxias commonly arise from genetic variants, which in children tend to be autosomal recessive conditions. It is imperative to consider treatable disorders. New genetic diagnostic techniques have emerged, enabling the identification of specific pathologies. However, a comprehensive description of the clinical and laboratory phenotypes of each patient is necessary to guide the genetic study and interpret the results. While there are currently limited treatable conditions, ongoing studies are proposing promising treatments for certain pathologies soon, thereby increasing the importance of accurate diagnostic approaches. Physical therapy is an important part of treatment. Occupational therapy, and speech or language therapy are also part of the symptomatic therapy.

Author details

Daniela Munoz Chesta* and Mónica Troncoso-Schifferli
Department of Pediatric Neurology, San Borja Arriaran Hospital, University of Chile, Santiago, Chile

*Address all correspondence to: daniela.munoz.c@uchile.cl

References

[1] Batten FE. Ataxia in childhood. Brain. 1905;**28**:484

[2] Konczak J, Timmann D. The effect of damage to the cerebellum on sensorimotor and cognitive function in children and adolescents. Neuroscience and Biobehavioral Reviews. 2007;**31**:1101-1113

[3] Musselman KE, Stoyanov CT, Marasigan R, et al. Prevalence of ataxia in children: A systematic review. Neurology. 2014;**82**:80-89

[4] Bernard G, Shevell M. The wobbly child: An approach to inherited ataxias. Seminars in Pediatric Neurology. 2008;**15**:194-208

[5] Winchester S et al. Ataxia. Handbook of Clinical Neurology. 2013;**112**:1213-1217. DOI: 10.1016/B978-0-444-52910-7.00043-X

[6] Pavone P, Praticò AD, Pavone V, et al. Ataxia in children: Early recognition and clinical evaluation. Italian Journal of Pediatrics. 2017;**43**:6

[7] Lynch DR, McCormick A, Schadt K, et al. Pediatric ataxia: Focus on chronic disorders. Seminars in Pediatric Neurology. 2018;**25**:54-64

[8] Prasad M, Ong MT, Setty G, et al. Fifteen-minute consultation: The child with acute ataxia. Archives of Disease in Childhood. Education and Practice Edition. 2013;**98**:217-223

[9] Gieron-Korthals MA, Westberry KR, Emmanuel PJ. Acute childhood ataxia: 10-year experience. Journal of Child Neurology. 1994;**9**:381-384

[10] Sirven JI, Fife TD, Wingerchuk DM, et al. Second-generation antiepileptic drugs' impact on balance: A meta-analysis. Mayo Clinic Proceedings. 2007;**82**:40-47

[11] Martínez González MJ, Martínez González S, García Ribes A, et al. Ataxia de aparición aguda en la infancia: etiología, tratamiento y seguimiento. Revista de Neurologia. 2006;**42**:321

[12] Akbar U, Ashizawa T. Ataxia. Neurologic Clinics. 2015;**33**:225-248

[13] van Gaalen J, Kerstens FG, Maas RPPWM, et al. Drug-induced cerebellar ataxia: A systematic review. CNS Drugs. 2014;**28**:1139-1153

[14] Whelan HT, Verma S, Guo Y, et al. Evaluation of the child with acute ataxia: A systematic review. Pediatric Neurology. 2013;**49**:15-24

[15] Connolly AM, Dodson WE, Prensky AL, et al. Course and outcome of acute cerebellar ataxia. Annals of Neurology. 1994;**35**:673-679

[16] Leake JAD, Albani S, Kao AS, et al. Acute disseminated encephalomyelitis in childhood: Epidemiologic, clinical and laboratory features. The Pediatric Infectious Disease Journal. 2004;**23**:756-764

[17] Banwell B, Kennedy J, Sadovnick D, et al. Incidence of acquired demyelination of the CNS in Canadian children. Neurology. 2009;**72**:232-239

[18] Cole J, Evans E, Mwangi M, et al. Acute disseminated encephalomyelitis in children: An updated review based on current diagnostic criteria. Pediatric Neurology. 2019;**100**:26-34

[19] Wang CX. Assessment and Management of Acute Disseminated Encephalomyelitis (ADEM) in the Pediatric patient. Pediatric Drugs. 2021;**23**:213-221

[20] Pavone P, Pettoello-Mantovano M, Le Pira A, et al. Acute disseminated encephalomyelitis: A long-term prospective study and meta-analysis. Neuropediatrics. 2010;**41**:246-255

[21] Shilo S, Michaeli O, Shahar E, et al. Long-term motor, cognitive and behavioural outcome of acute disseminated encephalomyelitis. European Journal of Paediatric Neurology. 2016;**20**:361-367

[22] Beatty C, Bowler RA, Farooq O, et al. Long-term neurocognitive, psychosocial, and magnetic resonance imaging outcomes in Pediatric-onset acute disseminated encephalomyelitis. Pediatric Neurology. 2016;**57**:64-73

[23] Brunklaus A, Pohl K, Zuberi SM, et al. Outcome and prognostic features in Opsoclonus-myoclonus syndrome from infancy to adult life. Pediatrics. 2011;**128**:e388-e394

[24] Galstyan A, Wilbur C, Selby K, et al. Opsoclonus-myoclonus syndrome: A new era of improved prognosis? Pediatric Neurology. 2017;**72**:65-69

[25] Blaes F, Dharmalingam B. Childhood opsoclonus-myoclonus syndrome: Diagnosis and treatment. Expert Review of Neurotherapeutics. 2016;**16**:641-648

[26] Cooper R, Khakoo Y, Matthay KK, et al. Opsoclonus-myoclonus-ataxia syndrome in neuroblastoma: Histopathologic features-a report from the children's cancer group. Medical and Pediatric Oncology. 2001;**36**:623-629

[27] Ostrom QT, Patil N, Cioffi G, et al. CBTRUS statistical report: Primary brain and other central nervous system Tumors diagnosed in the United States in 2013-2017. Neuro-oncology. 2020;**22**:iv1-iv96

[28] Rickert C, Paulus W. Epidemiology of central nervous system tumors in childhood and adolescence based on the new WHO classification. Child's Nervous System. 2001;**17**:503-511

[29] Aneja S, Sharma S. Diagnosis and Management of Acute Encephalitis in children. Indian Journal of Pediatrics. 2019;**86**:70-75

[30] Yeshokumar AK, Sun LR, Klein JL, et al. Gait disturbance as the presenting symptom in young children with anti-NMDA receptor encephalitis. Pediatrics. 2016;**138**:e20160901

[31] Baizabal-Carvallo JF, Stocco A, Muscal E, et al. The spectrum of movement disorders in children with anti-NMDA receptor encephalitis: Anti-Nmdar encephalitis movement disorders. Movement Disorders. 2013;**28**:543-547

[32] Goldberg EM, Titulaer M, de Blank PM, et al. Anti–N-methyl-D-aspartate receptor-mediated encephalitis in infants and toddlers: Case report and review of the literature. Pediatric Neurology. 2014;**50**:181-184

[33] Caffarelli M, Kimia AA, Torres AR. Acute ataxia in children: A review of the differential diagnosis and evaluation in the emergency department. Pediatric Neurology. 2016;**65**:14-30

[34] Overby P, Kapklein M, Jacobson RI. Acute ataxia in children. Pediatrics in Review. 2019;**40**:332-343

[35] Salman MS, Klassen SF, Johnston JL. Recurrent ataxia in children and

adolescents. Canadian Journal of Neurological Sciences. 2017;**44**:375-383

[36] Fernández-Alvarez E, Perez-Dueñas B. Paroxysmal movement disorders and episodic ataxias. Handbook of Clinical Neurology. 2013;**112**:847-852. DOI: 10.1016/B978-0-444-52910-7.00004-0

[37] Kipfer S, Strupp M. The clinical Spectrum of autosomal-dominant episodic ataxias. Movement Disorders Clinical Practice. 2014;**1**:285-290

[38] Garone G, Capuano A, Travaglini L, et al. Clinical and genetic overview of paroxysmal movement disorders and episodic ataxias. International Journal of Molecular Sciences. 2020;**21**:3603

[39] Jen JC, Wan J. Episodic ataxias. Handbook of Clinical Neurology. 2018;**148**:521-529. DOI: 10.1016/B978-0-444-64076-5.00033-8

[40] Koch H, Weber YG. The glucose transporter type 1 (Glut1) syndromes. Epilepsy & Behavior. 2019;**91**:90-93

[41] Gras D, Roze E, Caillet S, et al. GLUT1 deficiency syndrome: An update. Revue Neurologique (Paris). 2014;**170**:91-99

[42] Duat Rodriguez A, Prochazkova M, Santos Santos S, et al. Early diagnosis of CAPOS syndrome before acute-onset ataxia—Review of the literature and a new family. Pediatric Neurology. 2017;**71**:60-64

[43] Salles PA, Mata IF, Brünger T, et al. ATP1A3-related disorders: An ever-expanding clinical Spectrum. Frontiers in Neurology. 2021;**12**:637890

[44] Carecchio M, Zorzi G, Ragona F, et al. ATP1A3-related disorders: An update. European Journal of Paediatric Neurology. 2018;**22**:257-263

[45] Debray F-G, Lambert M, Gagne R, et al. Pyruvate dehydrogenase deficiency presenting as intermittent isolated acute ataxia. Neuropediatrics. 2008;**39**:20-23

[46] Pavuluri H, Alfiya F, Menon RN, et al. Pyruvate dehydrogenase complex deficiency due to PDHA1 mutation—A rare treatable cause for episodic ataxia in children. Indian Journal of Pediatrics. 2022;**89**:519-519

[47] Raslan IR, Barsottini OG, Pedroso JL. A proposed clinical classification and a diagnostic approach for congenital ataxias. Neurology: Clinical Practice. 2021;**11**:e328-e336

[48] Bertini E et al. Nonprogressive congenital ataxias. Handbook of Clinical Neurology. 2018;**155**:91-103. DOI: 10.1016/B978-0-444-64189-2.00006-8

[49] Correa GG, Amaral LF, Vedolin LM. Neuroimaging of Dandy-Walker malformation: New concepts. Topics in Magnetic Resonance Imaging. 2011;**22**:303-312

[50] Romani M, Micalizzi A, Valente EM. Joubert syndrome: Congenital cerebellar ataxia with the molar tooth. Lancet Neurology. 2013;**12**:894-905

[51] van Dijk T, Baas F, Barth PG, et al. What's new in pontocerebellar hypoplasia? An update on genes and subtypes. Orphanet Journal of Rare Diseases. 2018;**13**:92

[52] Soong B-W, Morrison PJ. Spinocerebellar ataxias. Handbook of Clinical Neurology. 2018; **155**:143-174. DOI: 10.1016/B978-0-444-64189-2.00010-X

[53] Beaudin M, Matilla-Dueñas A, Soong B-W, et al. The classification of autosomal recessive cerebellar ataxias: A consensus statement from the Society for Research on the cerebellum and ataxias task force. The Cerebellum. 2019;**18**:1098-1125

[54] Bürk K. Friedreich ataxia: Current status and future prospects. Cerebellum Ataxias. 2017;**4**:4

[55] Lecocq C, Charles P, Azulay J-P, et al. Delayed-onset Friedreich's ataxia revisited: The delayed-onset Friedreich's ataxia revisited. Movement Disorders. 2016;**31**:62-69

[56] Koeppen AH. Friedreich's ataxia: Pathology, pathogenesis, and molecular genetics. Journal of the Neurological Sciences. 2011;**303**:1-12

[57] Cook A, Giunti P. Friedreich's ataxia: Clinical features, pathogenesis and management. British Medical Bulletin. 2017;**124**:19-30

[58] Rothblum-Oviatt C, Wright J, Lefton-Greif MA, et al. Ataxia telangiectasia: A review. Orphanet Journal of Rare Diseases. 2016;**11**:159

[59] Teive HAG, Camargo CHF, Munhoz RP. More than ataxia – Movement disorders in ataxia-telangiectasia. Parkinsonism & Related Disorders. 2018;**46**:3-8

[60] Amirifar P, Ranjouri MR, Yazdani R, et al. Ataxia-telangiectasia: A review of clinical features and molecular pathology. Pediatric Allergy and Immunology. 2019;**30**:277-288

[61] Tang SY, Shaikh AG. Past and present of eye movement abnormalities in ataxia-telangiectasia. The Cerebellum. 2019;**18**:556-564

[62] Albaradie R, Alharbi A, Alsaffar G, et al. Ataxia with oculomotor apraxia type 1 associated with mutation in the APTX gene: A case study and literature review. Experimental and Therapeutic Medicine. 2022;**24**:709

[63] Liu W, Narayanan V. Ataxia with oculomotor apraxia. Seminars in Pediatric Neurology. 2008;**15**:216-220

[64] Anheim M, Monga B, Fleury M, et al. Ataxia with oculomotor apraxia type 2: Clinical, biological and genotype/phenotype correlation study of a cohort of 90 patients. Brain. 2009;**132**:2688-2698

[65] Tazir M, Ali-Pacha L, M'Zahem A, et al. Ataxia with oculomotor apraxia type 2: A clinical and genetic study of 19 patients. Journal of the Neurological Sciences. 2009;**278**:77-81

[66] Esmer C, Martínez AS, Palomo ER, et al. Hallazgos clínicos y moleculares en una paciente con ataxia por deficiencia de vitamina E, homocigota para la mutación c.205-1G>C en el gen TTPA. Boletín Médico del Hospital Infantil de México. 2013;**70**:6

[67] Muller DPR. Vitamin E and neurological function. Molecular Nutrition & Food Research. 2010;**54**:710-718

[68] Thapa S, Shah S, Chand S, Sah SK, Gyawali, P, Paudel S, et al. Ataxia due to vitamin E deficiency: A case report and updated review. Clinical Case Reports. 2022;**10**(9):e6303. DOI: 10.1002/ccr3.6303

[69] Xiromerisiou G, Dadouli K, Marogianni C, et al. A novel homozygous SACS mutation identified by whole exome sequencing-genotype phenotype correlations of all published cases. Journal of Molecular Neuroscience. 2020;**70**:131-141

[70] Bereznyakova O, Dupré N. Spastic ataxias. Handbook of Clinical Neurology. 2018;**155**:191-203. DOI: 10.1016/B978-0-444-64189-2.00012-3

[71] Vermeer S, Meijer RPP, Pijl BJ, et al. ARSACS in the Dutch population: A frequent cause of early-onset cerebellar ataxia. Neurogenetics. 2008;**9**:207-214

[72] Rezende Filho FM, Parkinson MH, Pedroso JL, et al. Clinical, ophthalmological, imaging and genetic features in Brazilian patients with ARSACS. Parkinsonism & Related Disorders. 2019;**62**:148-155

[73] Vill K, Müller-Felber W, Gläser D, et al. SACS variants are a relevant cause of autosomal recessive hereditary motor and sensory neuropathy. Human Genetics. 2018;**137**:911-919

[74] Patterson MC, Mengel E, Vanier MT, et al. Treatment outcomes following continuous miglustat therapy in patients with Niemann-pick disease type C: A final report of the NPC registry. Orphanet Journal of Rare Diseases. 2020;**15**:104

[75] Wheeler S, Sillence DJ. Niemann–pick type C disease: Cellular pathology and pharmacotherapy. Journal of Neurochemistry. 2020;**153**:674-692

[76] Vanier MT. Niemann-pick disease type C. Orphanet Journal of Rare Diseases. 2010;**5**:16

[77] Poujois A, Woimant F. Wilson's disease: A 2017 update. Clinics and Research in Hepatology and Gastroenterology. 2018;**42**:512-520

[78] Mulligan C, Bronstein JM. Wilson disease. Neurologic Clinics. 2020;**38**:417-432

[79] Członkowska A, Litwin T, Dusek P, et al. Wilson disease. Nature Reviews Disease Primers. 2018;**4**:21

[80] Pronk JC, van Kollenburg B, Scheper GC, et al. Vanishing white matter disease: A review with focus on its genetics. Mental Retardation and Developmental Disabilities Research Reviews. 2006;**12**:123-128

[81] Perez-Lloret S, Warrenburg B, Rossi M, et al. Assessment of ataxia rating scales and cerebellar functional tests: Critique and recommendations. Movement Disorders. 2021;**36**:283-297

[82] Sival DA, Brunt ER. The international cooperative ataxia rating scale shows strong age-dependency in children. Developmental Medicine and Child Neurology. 2009;**51**:571-572

[83] Lawerman TF, Brandsma R, Burger H, et al. Age-related reference values for the pediatric scale for assessment and rating of ataxia: A multicentre study. Developmental Medicine and Child Neurology. 2017;**59**:1077-1082

[84] Brandsma R, Spits AH, Kuiper MJ, et al. Ataxia rating scales are age-dependent in healthy children. Developmental Medicine and Child Neurology. 2014;**56**:556-563

[85] Brandsma R, Lawerman TF, Kuiper MJ, et al. Reliability and discriminant validity of ataxia rating scales in early onset ataxia. Developmental Medicine and Child Neurology. 2017;**59**:427-432

[86] Fonteyn EMR, Keus SHJ, Verstappen CCP, et al. The effectiveness of allied health care in patients with ataxia: A systematic review. Journal of Neurology. 2014;**261**:251-258

[87] Wang Y, Zhang D, Wang J, Ma J, Lu L, Jin S. Effects of transcranial magnetic stimulation on cerebellar ataxia: A systematic review and meta-analysis. Frontiers in Neurology. 2003;**14**:1049813. DOI: 10.3389/fneur.2023.1049813

[88] Chen TX, Yang C-Y, Willson G, et al. The efficacy and safety of transcranial direct current stimulation for cerebellar ataxia: A systematic review and meta-analysis. The Cerebellum. 2021;**20**:124-133

Chapter 4

Ataxia in Multiple Sclerosis: From Current Understanding to Therapy

Bilal El-Mansoury, Jawad Laadraoui, Abdelaati El Khiat, Omar El Hiba, Arumugam R. Jayakumar, Abdessalam Ferssiwi and Abdelali Bitar

Abstract

Ataxia is a type of neurological disorder that affects the ability to coordinate voluntary movements, such as walking, balance, and speech. In people with multiple sclerosis (MS), ataxia is a common symptom, affecting around 80% of people with the condition. The cause of ataxia in MS is still unknown; however, it is thought to be due to damage to the part of the central nervous system (CNS) that controls balance, coordination, and movement, especially the cerebellum. Symptoms of ataxia in people with MS can range from mild to severe, and can include a lack of coordination, difficulty speaking, difficulty walking, and gait. Ataxia management in MS typically involves pharmacotherapy to improve coordination, physiotherapy to enhance strength and balance, surgical procedures to alleviate tremor as well as occupational therapy to help with everyday activities.

Keywords: ataxia, tremor, multiple sclerosis, neurodegeneration, treatment

1. Introduction

Multiple sclerosis (MS) is an immune-mediated neurodegenerative disease of the central nervous system (CNS), which primary affects young adults [1–3]. The large immune response to putative CNS antigens is thought to be driven by an interplay between environmental and genetic factors [4]. There are four different forms of MS that can be distinguished based on the clinical disease pattern, namely: relapsing–remitting MS (RRMS), secondary progressive MS (SPMS), primary progressive MS (PPMS), and progressive relapsing MS (PRMS) [5]. Clinically, RRMS is the most common form of MS, with more than 85% of patients initially present with such form.

Multiple sclerosis is believed to be associated with a wide range of neurological abnormalities, which often interact to cause mobility difficulties, while the impairment in balance is thought to be significant factor in these mobility difficulties [6]. A body line of evidence shows that 85% of MS patients may experience mild ataxia at some point in time, while 32% of MS patients exhibits a severe form that can decline their functional abilities [7–9]. The word ataxia (from the Greek) literally means the

 IntechOpen

absence of order, disorder, or confusion and is characterized by a loss of coordination of the body's limbs, the trunk, and the gait and it can be brought on by sensory system's dysfunction (sensory ataxia), cerebellum's dysfunction (cerebellar ataxia), or dysfunction of the vestibular system (vestibular ataxia) [10, 11], which may also arise from thalamic and parietal- and frontal-lobe injuries [8].

Clinically, ataxia refers to a collection of abnormal movements, of which tremor is the main symptom. Other clinical manifestations include dysmetria, dysdiadochokinesia, incoordination, and movement delays [8]. It is rarely seen as a single symptom and usually occurs with muscle weakness and spasticity [7]. Nevertheless, severe ataxia may occur alone but it is usually combined with brainstem signs [12]. A range of interventions aimed at enhancing balance in standing and walking are used in clinical practice, including pharmacotherapy, surgical therapies, and the most common is physiotherapy. This chapter provides an overview of different types of ataxia, the current understanding of ataxia in MS, and the currently available therapeutic approaches.

2. Clinical features of cerebellar dysfunction in MS

Cerebellar dysfunction is a typical feature of MS, which results in a wide range of neurological manifestations. The clinical signs of cerebellar involvement in MS include gait ataxia, dysmetria when performing the finger-to-nose and heel-to-shin tests, and the inability to perform tandem gait [4]. Cerebellar involvement in MS results from both vermian and hemispheric lesions. Up to 50% of MS patients may experience intention tremor and limb ataxia [4]. Indeed, MS frequently causes coordination issues, which are mostly brought on by pathology in the cerebellum itself or dysfunction in cerebellar connections, including proprioceptive afferent inputs. Depending on the exact location of the lesion, cerebellar dysfunction can cause limb, gait, and truncal ataxia as well as other cerebellar characteristics including dysarthria, and tremor [13]. MS patients exhibit signs of either chronic cerebellar abnormalities in a progressing disease or acute cerebellar impairment related to an acute relapse [13]. A higher incidence of cerebellar involvement during successive relapses appears to be linked to cerebellar relapse in the early stages of the disease [14].

It is believed that injury to the anterior lobe of the cerebellum is the primary cause of gait ataxia [15]. Cerebellar dysarthria is a rare symptom at disease initiation but is common in people with secondary progressive diseases that have worsened [13]. Although paroxysmal MS symptoms are rare, paroxysmal dysarthria with ataxia has been documented in MS and is thought to be related to midbrain pathology [16, 17]. Sensory evaluation (sensory ataxia) based on as scoring from 0 to 4, shows minimal sensory impairment in MS patients. The minimal sensory impairment detected clinically was found to be more prominent in the electrophysiological studies [7].

A recent database research of over 15,000 patients found that there were nearly 50,000 total relapses. Cerebellar relapses made up about 10% of those, and they were more common in men and in people who had had the disease for a longer period of time [18]. Poor relapse recovery is also linked to cerebellar/brainstem relapses, which are linked to an earlier onset of progressive disease [13].

Likewise, tremor is a common symptom of MS and has been found in more than half of MS patients who visit specialized clinics [11]. Clinical studies have revealed that tremor was clinically detected in 18 MS patients and absent in 14 patients. While

MS patients who had a visible tremor had an ataxia score that was more severe and showed clinical symptoms of cerebellar dysfunction [19]. It is worth mentioning that cerebellar ataxia is generally associated with tremor, which typically happens during voluntary movements or while maintaining a position [11]. MS tremor is believed to be mostly brought on by cerebellar and/or thalamic dysfunction [20]. Otherwise, tremor can occur in the head, limbs, vocal cords, and trunk. Though rest and rubral tremors are uncommon, intention and postural tremors are the most prevalent types [21, 22]. Whereas, severe tremor, which is thought to affect 3% of MS patients, is a very uncommon but severely debilitating MS complication [22]. The pathophysiology of tremor in MS is complex and is thought to involve connections between the cerebellum, cerebral cortex, and basal ganglia [13]. Given the significance of cerebellar connections in motor control, it may not be surprising that the involvement of the cerebellum is associated with higher impairment and a worse prognosis.

3. Classification of ataxia

Based on the location, there are different forms of ataxia: cerebellar, sensory, and vestibular ataxia. It can be further divided into three categories: acquired (caused by structural or demyelinating conditions, toxicity, paraneoplastic, inflammatory or infectious diseases, and autoimmune conditions), hereditary (caused by a gene defect and manifesting in childhood), and sporadic (patients have no family history of ataxia and present in adulthood) [23]. The most prevalent of the genetic types of ataxias is Friedreich's ataxia (FRDA), which is autosomal recessive.

3.1 Primary ataxia

Ataxias that affect the primary cerebellum can also be considered as sporadic and inherited. The latter includes episodic ataxias, X-linked cerebellar ataxias, mitochondrial ataxias, autosomal dominant cerebellar ataxias, also known as spinocerebellar ataxias (SCAs), and autosomal recessive cerebellar ataxias (ARCAs). The cerebellar variant of multiple system atrophy (MSA-C) and idiopathic late-onset cerebellar ataxias are examples of idiopathic degenerative cerebellar ataxias [24–31].

3.2 Congenital ataxia

Cerebellar malformations or pontocerebellar hypoplasia can produce congenital ataxias, which manifest as cerebellar ataxias. The uncommon autosomal recessive condition, Joubert's syndrome, whose most well-known manifestation is the "molar tooth sign" on MRI, is defined by a congenital hind-brain abnormality. The clinical picture includes multiple organ involvement, cerebellar ataxia, respiratory dysregulation, ocular motor apraxia, and neonatal hypotonia. Till now, more than 20 causal genes have been found, the majority of which encode proteins for the main cilium, and an organelle found within cells that plays a key role in many cellular processes. The genetic condition known as ciliopathies, which is a new class, includes Joubert's syndrome (**Figure 1**) [32, 33].

3.3 Inherited ataxia

The vast set of clinically and genetically diverse, complicated neurodegenerative disorders known as inherited cerebellar ataxias is brought on by several genetic

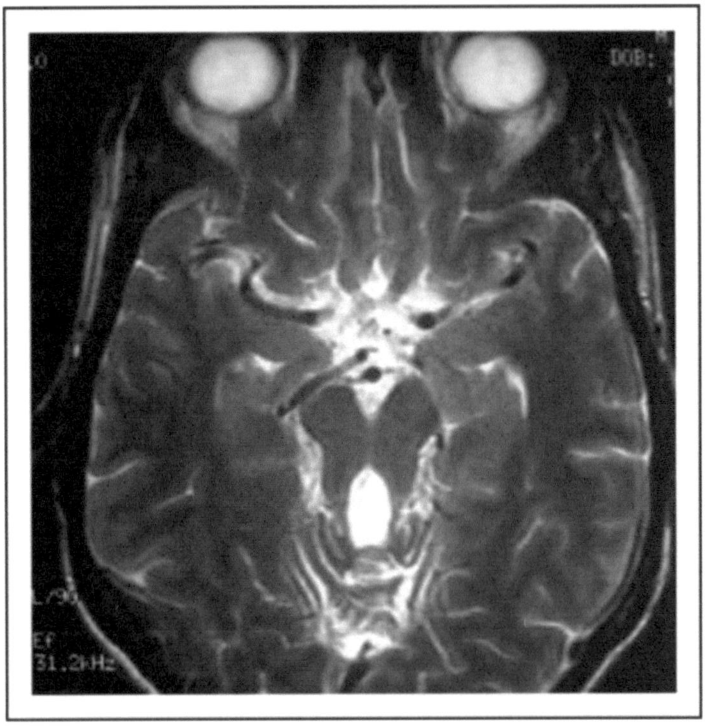

Figure 1.
T2-weighted, axial image of a brain MRI in a patient presenting Joubert's syndrome and the molar tooth sign [23].

abnormalities. There are two X-linked ataxias, more than 30 ARCAs, almost 40 SCA forms, and several mitochondrial ataxias among the hereditary cerebellar ataxias [24, 25, 31, 34].

3.4 Mitochondrial ataxia

Cerebellar and sensory ataxias, which are caused by defects in mitochondrial DNA, are frequently coupled with additional symptoms in mitochondrial ataxias [35]. These ataxias include maternally inherited hereditary ataxias caused by deletions or duplications of mitochondrial DNA or point mutations in the genes encoding for RNAs and respiratory chain components [35, 36]. A mutation in the mitochondrial DNA polymerase subunit gamma (POLG) gene results in mitochondrial recessive ataxia syndrome [35, 36]. With cerebellar and afferent/sensory ataxia, POLG-related ataxia is a mixed ataxia that manifests with a variety of non-ataxia symptoms, including sensory neuropathy, external ophthalmoplegia, ptosis, epilepsy, and hyperkinetic movement abnormalities [35, 36].

3.5 Idiopathic degenerative ataxia

As well as being referred to as sporadic adult-onset ataxia (SAOA) of unknown etiology or even idiopathic sporadic cerebellar ataxia, MSA-C and idiopathic late-onset cerebellar ataxia are two examples of the diseases with unknown etiology that fall within the category of idiopathic cerebellar degeneration [26, 27, 29, 30, 37, 38].

3.6 Secondary ataxia

Ataxias caused by exogenous or endogenous nongenetic factors, such as those that are toxic, paraneoplastic, immune-mediated, nutritional, and infectious in character, as well as localized damage to the cerebellum, fall under the category of secondary or acquired ataxias [26, 29, 30]. When characterizing localized lesions in the cerebellum and its connections due to conditions including neoplastic, inflammatory, demyelinating, and vascular illnesses, neuroimaging investigations are crucial [26, 29, 30]. The unfavorable effects of some medications might also cause ataxia [39]. Whereas, antiepileptic drugs like oxcarbazepine, lamotrigine, and phenytoin, benzodiazepines like nitrazepam and triazolam, and antineoplastic/immunosuppressive medications like cytarabine, tacrolimus, and cyclosporine are the most prevalent causes of drug-induced cerebellar ataxia [39]. Ataxia can also be brought on by chemicals including alcohol, lithium, and toluene [39, 40]. Otherwise, cerebellar ataxia can result from a number of infectious diseases, including syphilis, Whipple's disease, the mumps, and infectious mononucleosis [26, 29, 30]. It can also be a symptom of endocrine disorders, notably hypothyroidism. Hashimoto's encephalopathy, also known as a steroid-responsive encephalopathy, is associated with autoimmune thyroiditis (Thomas [26, 29, 30]). Whereas, it has been reported that people who do not get enough vitamins including thiamine, tocopherol, and cobalamin may develop cerebellar and afferent/sensory ataxias [26, 29, 30]. While antibodies against glutamic acid decarboxylase (GAD), which were first identified in individuals with stiff-person syndrome, have also been linked to cerebellar ataxia [26, 29, 30, 41, 42]. A body of evidence sustain a sex dimorphism of such immune-mediated cerebellum condition, with women being more likely to have anti-GAD ataxia, which can also coexist with thyroid disorders and insulin-dependent diabetic mellitus. While intravenous immunoglobulins and steroids have varying effects on anti-GAD ataxia. Otherwise, gluten ataxia is another immune-mediated condition brought on by gluten consumption in people with a genetic predisposition [43]. The disease is characterized by adult-onset, progressive gait ataxia with gaze-evoked nystagmus and peripheral neuropathy symptoms. In all cases, the anti-gliadin antibody is positive and an anti-gluten diet can enhance gluten ataxia [43].

3.7 Autosomal recessive cerebellar ataxia

Autosomal recessive cerebellar ataxias (ARCAs) are a part of the diverse category of hereditary ataxias. They often start young and are marked by degeneration of the cerebellum and spinal cord [24, 26, 29–31]. **Table 1** displays the most typical ARCAs that have been genetically identified, wherein we note that ataxia telangiectasia and FRDA are the two most prevalent forms in white children [24, 31, 44, 45].

3.8 Friedreich's ataxia

Since the identification of the FRDA gene and the GAA trinucleotide expansion that causes FRDA, phenotypic variants of this ataxia have been regularly reported in individuals with pathogenic mutations [44, 46]. Some of these variations do not correspond to how this sickness is usually described. Atypical phenotypes include movement abnormalities, pyramidal signals, preserved reflexes, late-onset and very-late-onset ataxia, minor GAA expansions, and ataxia [47, 48].

Autosomal recessive cerebellar ataxia types	Locus	Gene	Protein
Friedreich's ataxia	9q13	*FXN*	Frataxin
Ataxia with vitamin E deficiency	8q12.3	*TTPA*	α-Tocopherol transfer protein
Autosomal recessive spastic cerebellar ataxia of Charlevoix-Saguenay	13q12	*SACS*	Sacsin
Ataxia telangiectasia	11q22.3	*ATM*	Serine protein kinase
Ataxia telangiectasia-like disorder	11q21	*MRE11*	Meiotic recombination 11
Ataxia with oculomotor apraxia type 1	9p13	*APTX*	Aprataxin
Ataxia with oculomotor apraxia type 2	9q34	*SETX*	Senataxin
Mitochondrial recessive ataxia syndrome	15q25	*POLG1*	DNA polymerase subunit g-1
Marinesco-Sjogren syndrome	5q31	*SIL1*	Nucleotide exchange factor SIL1
Autosomal recessive cerebellar ataxia type 1	6q25	*SYNE1*	Nesprin-1
Autosomal recessive cerebellar ataxia type 2	1q42.2	*CABC1*	Chaperone activity of bc1 complex like
Autosomal recessive cerebellar ataxia type 3	3p22.1	*ANO10*	Anoctamin-10

Table 1.
The most prevalent kinds of autosomal recessive cerebellar ataxias with genetic definition.

Friedreich's ataxia is largely an ataxia of the efferent and sensory nerves where neuropathological investigations and more recent neuroimaging studies have both verified the existence of a cerebellar component (**Figure 2**) [44, 46, 49]. Nevertheless, antioxidants like coenzyme Q10 and its derivatives, such as idebenone, have been employed, despite the lack of agreement on a cure. Although it is ineffective for neurological disorders, idebenone has demonstrated notable advantages for hypertrophic cardiomyopathy [50, 51]. Deferiprone and epigenetic treatment for Friedreich's ataxia have both recently undergone testing, as have other novel medications [52, 53].

3.9 Ataxia telangiectasia

More than 200 potentially harmful mutations affecting virtually all of the ataxia telangiectasia-mutated (ATM) gene's coding exons have been identified since the ATM gene was initially characterized [54]. In addition to the typical phenotype with cerebellar ataxia and oculocutaneous telangiectasia, many instances of ataxia telangiectasia with milder phenotypes have been documented (**Figure 3**). These phenotypes involve later diagnosis, lower progression of the disease, longer life expectancy, an affinity for movement disorders such as dystonia, myoclonus, and chorea instead of cerebellar ataxia, an absence of ocular telangiectasia, decreased levels of chromosomal instability and cellular radiosensitivity, as well as the absence of ocular telangiectasia [45, 54]. Actually, ataxia telangiectasia is a multisystem disorder with a range of neurological and systemic symptoms. A more appropriate name for this condition has been suggested: as ATM syndrome.

3.10 Spinocerebellar ataxia

Spinocerebellar ataxias (SCAs) are a sizable and intricate collection of diverse autosomal dominant degenerative illnesses that affect several parts of the

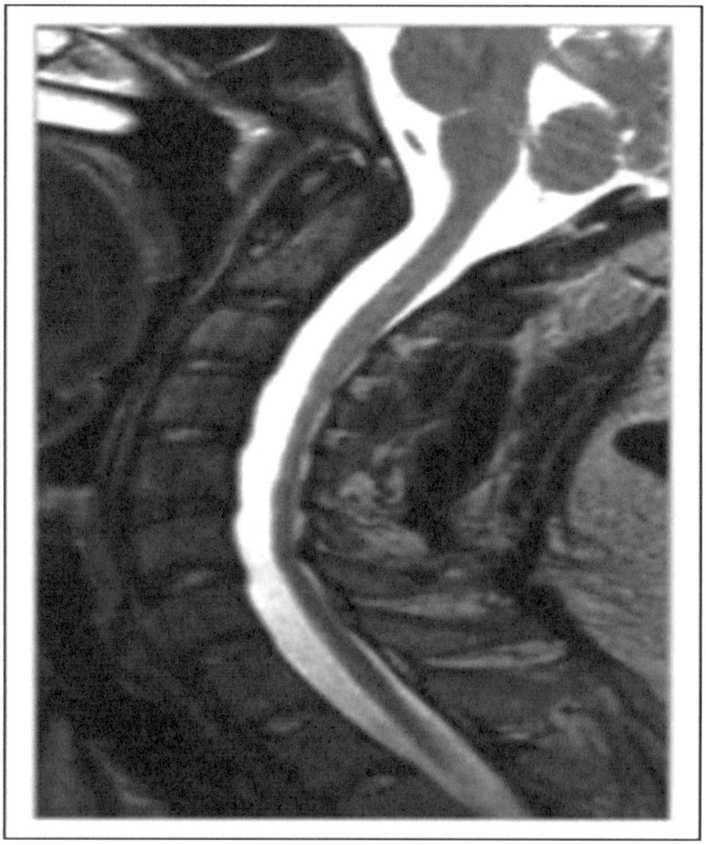

Figure 2.
Sagittal image of a T2-weighted MRI of the spinal cord of patient presenting Friedreich's ataxia with cervical spinal cord atrophy [23].

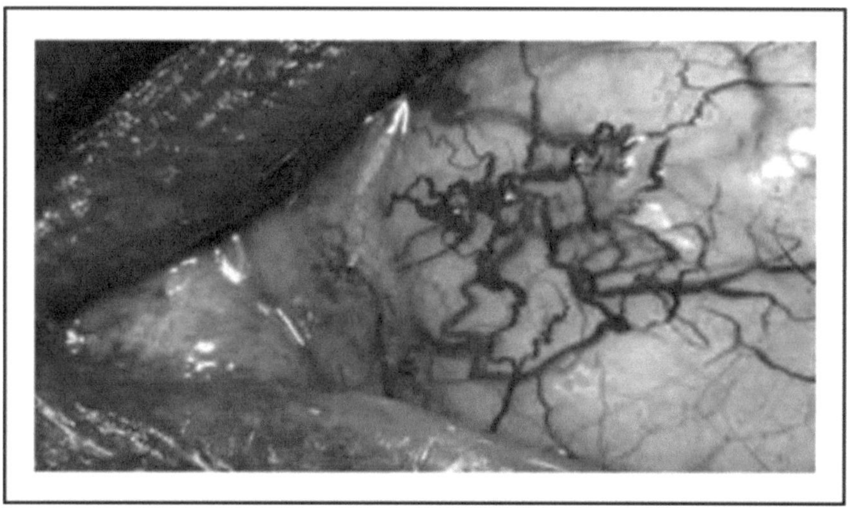

Figure 3.
A patient with ataxia telangiectasia with conjunctival telangiectasia [23].

neurological system, including the cerebellum and its efferent and afferent connections [25, 26, 28–30, 34, 55–57]. **Table 2** lists the most common SCA subtypes along with the genetic locations, mutations, and proteins linked to each condition from SCA type 1 through SCA type 40. The most prevalent form of SCA is type 3, while types 1, 2, 6, and 7 have significantly different prevalence depending on the racial makeup of the population [25–30, 34, 57]. The genetic etiology of illness is still unknown in roughly 40–50% of ARCAs, despite great progress in the discovery of ARCA genes [58–64]. With the exception of ataxia brought on by a vitamin E shortage and a set of ataxias linked to a coenzyme Q10 deficiency, there is no known therapy for these ataxias [26, 29, 30, 58, 63].

Entity	Locus	Gene	Mutation	Potential identifying clinical characteristics
SCA1 (spinocerebellar ataxia type 1)	6p22–23	*ATXN1*	CAG expansion	Hypermetric saccades, corticospinal tract signs
SCA2	12q23–24.1	*ATXN2*	CAG expansion	Slow saccades, areflexia
SCA3 (Machado-Joseph diseases)	14q32.1	*ATXN3/ DMJ*	CAG expansion	Bulging eyes, fasciculations
SCA4	16q22.1	*SCA4*		
SCA5	11q13.2	*SPTBN2*	Deletion, point mutation	Downbeat nystagmus
SCA6	19p13	*CACNA1A*	CAG expansion	Coarse nystagmus and saccadic intrusions
SCA7	3p21.1-p12	*ATXN7*	CAG expansion	Visual loss due to retinal degeneration
SCA8	13q21	*ATXN8OS*	CAG/CTG expansion	Reduced penetrance
SCA10	22q13.31	*ATXN10*	ATTCT expansion	Seizures
SCA11	15q15.2	*TTBK2*	Deletion	Downbeat nystagmus
SCA12	5q32	*PPP2R2B*	CAG expansion	Action tremor in midlife
SCA13	19q13.33	*KCNC3*	Point mutation	Absent eye findings
SCA14	19q13.4	*PRKCG*	Deletion, point mutation	Tremor, myoclonus, facial myokymia
SCA15/ SCA16	3p26.1	*ITPR1*	Duplication	Postural and kinetic tremor, psychiatric symptoms or dementia
SCA17	6q27	*TBP*	CAG	Huntington's disease like (dysarthria before gait ataxia)
SCA20	11p11.2-q13.3	*SCA20*	Multiple gene duplication	Spasmodic dysphonia, palatal tremor
SCA27	13q34	*FGF14*	Point mutation	Mental retardation and tremor
SCA28	18p11	*AFG3L2*	Point mutation	
SCA29	3p26.1	*ITPR1*	Allelic to SCA15, 16	Congenital nonprogressive ataxia

Entity	Locus	Gene	Mutation	Potential identifying clinical characteristics
SCA30	4q34.3-q35.1	*SCA30*		
SCA31	16q22	*SCA31*	TGGAA	
SCA32	7q32-q33	*SCA32*		
SCA34	6q12.3-q16.1	*AFG3L2*	Point mutation	Erythrokeratodermia
SCA35	20p13	*TGM6*		
SCA36	20p13	*NOP56*	GGCCTG expansion	Myoclonus, choreoathetosis, dementia (Huntington's disease like)
SCA37	1p32	*SCA37*		
SCA38	6p12.1	*ELOVLE5*		
SCA40	14q32	*CCDC88C*		
Dentatorubral-pallidoluysian atrophy (DRPLA)	12p13.31	*ATN1*	CAG expansion	Hyperkeratosis, multiple system atrophy-cerebellar type-like (Huntington's disease like)
Episodic ataxia type 1		*KCNA1*		Episodic, lasts seconds to minutes, interictal fasciculations
Episodic ataxia type 1		*CACNA1Q*		Episodic, lasts from hours to days, interictal nystagmus

Table 2.
Genetic characteristics of spinocerebellar ataxias.

Other SCAs cover a wide range of clinical symptoms. As opposed to the normal phenotype, which comprises of cerebellar ataxia and epilepsy, the major phenotype seen in the latter is pure cerebellar [29, 30]. It is worth mentioning that several additional SCAs with novel loci and gene mutations have been described more recently and SCA patients have a relatively high number of mutations, however, many patients (30–40%) still lack a genetic or molecular diagnosis [34, 57].

3.11 Secondary ataxias

Secondary or acquired ataxias include ataxias arising from exogenous or endogenous nongenetic origins, including those naturally caused toxins, paraneoplastic, immune-mediated agents, and infections, as well as focal injury to the cerebellum [26, 65, 66]. In MS, inflammation attacks and damages nerve fibers and myelin, a protective tissue around the nerves of the brain and spinal cord. Eventually, nerve cells that control body movements by sending and receiving electrical signals are damaged, which leads to abnormalities in body movement. In patients with MS, three types of ataxias are cerebellar, sensory (proprioceptive ataxia), and vestibular ataxia. Cerebellar ataxia is a syndrome that encompasses gait ataxia, nystagmus, dysarthria, tremor, and cognitive dysfunction, among others [67]. It is caused by damage to the cerebellum, leading to disruptions in the actions of different nerves that control muscle and movements on one or both sides of the body. Vestibular ataxia causes loss of balance, vertigo, dizziness, nausea, and vomiting, among others. Some people with

MS develop vestibular ataxia slowly, so they just have a loss of balance or equilibrium, not other severe symptoms. Vestibular ataxia is caused by damage to the vestibular system (i.e., inner ear structures and fluid-filled ear canals that control the sense of balance) and it might also be caused by lesions in the brainstem, or if MS pathology affects nerves that connect tiny organs in the inner ear that control balance. In this setting, neuroimaging studies are of great importance in determining focal lesions in the cerebellum and its connections as well as other affected parts of the brain [67].

4. Diagnosing patients with ataxia

The history should provide information on the kind of ataxia or vestibular dysfunction, the body areas affected, any concomitant signs, and the underlying etiology. Neurologists will be able to anticipate the results of the physical examination with a high degree of accuracy if they take a thorough history. Any unexpected physical discoveries should be cause for rethinking the past.

Numerous concomitant signs and symptoms of ataxia may appear, allowing the neurologist to focus on the differential diagnosis. Postural problems in case of cerebellar ataxia can be assessed objectively and subjectively. An accurate assessment of clinical symptoms serves as the foundation for qualitative evaluations. Cerebellar ataxia is indicated by postural instability and a stumbling, jerky gait. Since instruction regarding gait and gait disorders is rarely given much attention in medical colleges, an accurate examination of clinical symptoms is frequently overlooked [68].

- **Mental status examination:** There is growing understanding of the cerebellum's function in cognition. Along with being the location of motor coordination, the cerebellum also interacts closely with the cerebrum to perform higher-order cortical tasks, such as frontal executive functions, spatial orientation, motor memory, language skills, and the ability to recognize and express emotions [68].

- **Cranial nerve examination:** Examining extraocular movements typically shows aberrant pursuit and saccades, ocular dyskinesia such as square-wave jerks, ocular flutter, and opsoclonus in a variety of cerebellar illnesses. A cerebellar mass lesion may cause papilledema, particularly in people with hydrocephalus. The ipsilateral loss of the corneal reflex and impairment of the eighth cranial nerve may be signs of a cerebellopontine angle tumor. SCA3 symptoms include facial and tongue fasciculations, and SCA36 symptoms include significant tongue atrophy and fasciculations.

- **Vestibular signs:** The majority of the time, ataxia from the vestibular system is accompanied by vertigo and sluggish nystagmus with or without change in posture. When trying to walk straight, affected patients frequently deviate to the ipsilateral side. To rule out problems with the inner ear, hearing loss should be further assessed.

- **Cerebellar signs:** Often, the gait is impacted first. They are unable to stand with their feet together. Walking or adopting a tandem posture is a more sensitive test. Patients frequently lean in the same direction. With titubation, the gait is wide based. A localized cerebellar lesion frequently causes dysmetria of the limbs, intention tremor, loss of control, hypotonia, and dorsal spooning (hyperextension of interphalangeal joints) of the hand, in addition to dysarthria and nystagmus. In addition to appendicular ataxia, which should be assessed by looking at limb movements, and upright ataxia, which should be assessed by looking at posture, gait, and truncal ataxia, physical examinations should also look for ocular dyskinesias, speech abnormalities, proprioceptive loss, and vestibular dysfunction.

- **Extrapyramidal symptoms:** It is typical for extrapyramidal symptoms to be accompanied by persistently increasing ataxia. Extrapyramidal symptoms are frequently a clue that a neurodegenerative process is moving beyond the cerebellum and brainstem in inherited ataxias. For instance, whereas MSA and certain SCAs may also have linked Parkinsonism, most SCAs often impact gait first. Levodopa frequently alleviates the symptoms of Parkinsonism in SCA2, SCA3, and SCA17; however, when the striatum is affected, patients frequently have Parkinsonism and are not sensitive to levodopa. In these individuals receiving levodopa medication, dyskinesia can be brought on; nevertheless, involuntary movements, including dystonia, may be a symptom of SCAs. To find them, the inspection may need careful attention.

- **Strength:** It is critical to determine whether muscular weakness may account for the severity of ataxia. The examiner might ask the patient to rise up from a sitting posture and to stand on their toes and heels in order to assess the functional proximal and distal muscular strength while compensating for ataxia. Myopathy is suggested by symmetrically proximal muscle weakness. Generalized neuropathy is suggested by distal muscular weakness. In addition to ataxia, muscular weakness may also be indicated by abnormal gait. For instance, waddling gait, which should not be confused with ataxic gait, is caused when the hip girdle is weak owing to myopathy, which causes the pelvis to have a tendency to move toward the side.

- **Proprioceptive sensory system:** Sensory ataxia may result from a loss of sensory information from spinocerebellar pathways to the cerebellum. Any proprioceptive pathway impairment, including Friedreich's ataxia, ataxia with vitamin E deficiency, acquired sensory ataxias linked to ataxic polyneuropathies (e.g., paraneoplastic sensory neuronopathy), Sjögren's syndrome, diabetes mellitus, vitamin B6 toxicity, and Miller Fisher syndrome, may result in sensory loss. Proprioception and vibration at the great toe can be used to evaluate this. In contrast to cerebellar ataxia, where there is no change in the severity of ataxia with and without the eyes closed, the ataxia often gets worse when the visual signals are removed. Additionally, these individuals struggle to stand with their feet together and their eyes closed (Romberg sign).

5. Neuroanatomy and neuropathology of ataxia

Ataxia is a condition that affects the cerebellum and its afferent and efferent connections, the vestibular system, and the proprioceptive sensory pathway (**Figure 4**). The cerebellum is often divided into the cerebellar hemispheres and the midline cerebellum. A separate form of ataxia may manifest after lesions in any of these areas. For instance, injury to the unilateral cerebellar hemisphere typically results in ipsilateral cerebellar ataxia, whereas damage to the midline cerebellar structures typically manifests as gait impairment and truncal ataxia.

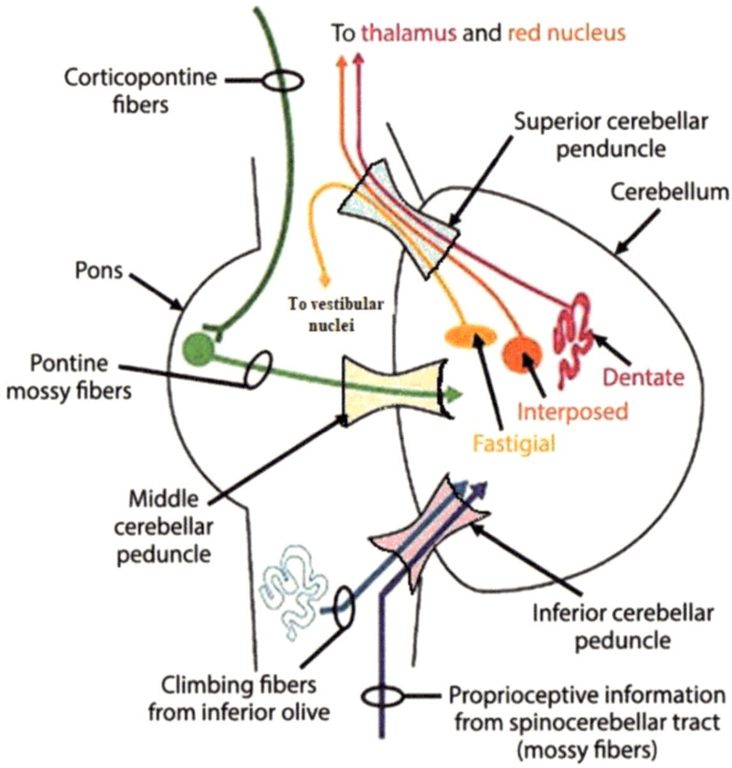

Figure 4.
The cerebellum's afferent and efferent connections. Climbing fibers from the inferior olives pass through the inferior cerebellar peduncles to link to the cerebellum, whereas pontine mossy fibers pass through the middle cerebellar peduncles. The superior cerebellar peduncles receive cerebellar outputs from the dentate nucleus and other deep cerebellar nuclei.

A lesion that disrupts the sensory transmission to the cerebellum may be the cause of ataxia. Spinal ataxia or sensory ataxia may result from this disease. Cerebellar ataxia is brought on by a break in the cerebellum's cortical impulses. Both of the aforementioned disorders can lead to spinocerebellar ataxias. They are caused by chromosomal CAG repetition and are autosomal dominant. Characteristic findings vary depending on where the lesion is located and include:

- Diffuse lesions result in widespread symptoms, whereas lesions in the lateral cerebellum only induce symptoms on the side of the lesion (ipsilateral).
- Ataxia of the limbs is brought on by cerebellar hemisphere lesions.
- Truncal, gait ataxia is caused by vermis lesions that spare the limbs.
- Vertigo, imbalance, and gait ataxia are all symptoms of vestibulo-cerebellar lesions, chromosomes [69].

Localization can be aided by comprehension of this neuroanatomy and its relationship to coordination. Despite the fact that there is considerable clinical overlap among them, the relationships are presented in **Table 3**.

Neuroanatomy	Function	Ataxia or ataxia-like presentation arising from damage of the region
Cerebellar hemisphere, including dentate nuclei	combining motor planning with sensory information to coordinate difficult tasks	Ipsilateral limb ataxia, dysdiadochokinesia, dysmetria, intention tremor, and scanning speech
Midline cerebellar structures (vermis, fastigial and interposed nuclei, the vestibulocerebellum, and the paravermis)	Balance, coordination of the lower extremities, fast and slow eye movements, and vestibular function	Gait ataxia and imbalance, truncal ataxia, dysmetria, ocular findings, head bobbing, and vertigo
Posterior lobe (flocculonodular lobe)	including information on vestibular nuclei	Nystagmus, postural instability, and gait ataxia
Cerebral cortex (frontal lobe)	Planning and initiating gait	Frontal ataxia (Bruns apraxia), magnetic gait (not the same as ataxic gait), although damage in this area that is related to the ataxia might make it worse.
Brainstem (vestibular nuclei, inferior olivary nuclei, pontine nuclei, and cerebellar peduncles)	Relay signals in and out of the cerebellum	Ataxia associated with cranial nerve dysfunction and motor-sensory deficits
Spinal cord (cuneate fasciculus, gracile fasciculus, and spinocerebellar tracts [mossy fibers])	Sensory pathways conduction	Sensory ataxia
Musculoskeletal system (gluteal muscles)	Stabilizing the weight-bearing hip	Waddling gait rather than ataxia, however disease in this area that is connected to it can make ataxia worse
Peripheral sensation system and visual system	Proprioception, visual cues	Sensory ataxia with Romberg sign, can worsen cerebellar ataxia
Vestibular system (labyrinth of the inner ear, vestibular nerve, and vestibular nuclei)	Sense of balance and special orientation, equilibrium	Unsteadiness, loss of balance brought on by vertigo, and a feeling of heaviness, tinnitus, and hearing loss, as well as nystagmus

Table 3.
Clinical characteristics and neuroanatomical relationships in ataxia.

6. Management of ataxia in MS

Management of ataxia and tremor encompasses a variety of available treatments, ranging from pharmacological approaches, surgical strategies to neurorehabilitation [10, 70]. The effectiveness and safety of treatments for ataxia in MS are not well understood; however, neurosurgery and rehabilitation procedures may be at least somewhat helpful [8]. Ataxia and tremor are challenging symptoms for management and treatments are supportive only [10, 11, 71]. Broadly speaking, the management of MS is based either on symptomatic treatments for established symptoms and/or disease-modifying therapies (DMTs), which aim to alleviate the impact of this condition [13].

Surgical procedures like deep brain stimulation (DBS) may be useful for some patients and prior to invasive procedures, a team examination of each individual is necessary [10]. The most popular non-pharmacological treatment for MS ataxia is physiotherapy, which is used frequently. Exercises designed specifically for balance that facilitate somatosensory and motor strategies are typically used, albeit to various degrees [72]. Task-oriented training also improves ambulation and postural control in MS patients by fostering motor learning [73]. Combinations of these physiotherapy techniques are generally considered to be highly beneficial for MS patients [74].

Finding new treatment approaches will be aided by a better understanding of the pathophysiology of cerebellar disease in MS which will help to treat its related ataxia and tremor. Hence, treating cerebellar disorders and offering neuroprotection inside the cerebellum are urgently needed while newer treatments are being tested, like stem cell therapy. The possibility of stem cell therapies for MS cerebellar pathology is particularly alluring, given the revelation that Purkinje cell fusion is a potential neurorestorative mechanism [13]. A summary of treatment modalities and options for the ataxia of MS patients is provided in **Table 4** [75–77].

6.1 Pharmacological treatment

Pharmacological treatment for cerebellar ataxia also remains challenging. Case report studies and small studies offer little support for certain treatments. Although recommendations are difficult to make for the treatment of ataxia and tremor, a variety of medications have been shown to have advantages in small open-label studies or case reports. Several treatments have been used including propranolol [78], isoniazid [76, 77], topiramate [79], carbamazepine [80], clonazepam, and levetiracetam [81] and reported only little success [10]. In a small pilot research involving 14 MS patients, levetiracetam was also found to dramatically lessen tremor and ataxia [82]. Moreover, topiramate has shown significant functional improvement in a sustained, dose-dependent manner [79]. Additionally, fingolimod may have added benefits in MS patients with ataxia [75]. Other drugs tested including glutethimide [83], cannabinoids [84], and dolasetron mesylate [85]. Cannabis extracts have been the subject of several randomized controlled trials, and the results have shown that cannabinoids do not seem to reduce MS tremor [84, 86, 87]. There is some evidence that paroxysmal ataxia and dysarthria may respond to carbamazepine in a manner comparable to other paroxysmal symptoms of MS, such as tonic spasm [88].

Although isoniazid, propranolol, and levetiracetam have been investigated, the findings are inconclusive, and these drugs are not frequently used (the patients included in these trials were typically very small, allowing for few generalizations) [76, 78, 81, 89–91]. Whereas, isoniazide in high doses, carbamazepine, propranolol,

Treatment Modality	Options
Physical	Balance-based torso weighting, task oriented, and core-stability exercises
Pharmacologic therapy	Carbamazepine, topiramate, Isoniazide, levetracetam, phenytoin, acetazolamide, lacosamide, fingolimod[#]
Surgical approches[*]	Deep brain stimulation, thalamotomy

[*]*Adverse effects such as dysarthria and ataxia disability scores not improved.*
[#]*To be used with caution as it has significant immunosuppressive effects.*

Table 4.
Treatment modalities and options for the ataxia of multiple sclerosis (MS) patients.

glutethimide, 4-aminopyridine, and topiramate have been reported to provide some benefit in the treatment of ataxia and tremor [20, 79, 92]. As ataxia constitutes a difficult symptom to treat, medications like isoniazid and carbamezepine must be used in high amounts for the treatment to be effective. Since these medications have hepatotoxic effects, many patients are unable to receive the maximum dosage, which limits their ability to be used for extended periods of time [7]. Indeed, pharmacological approaches used to improve ataxic symptoms are generally disappointing, necessitating the need for innovative treatments. In a meta-analysis study performed by Mills et al. [70], the authors have reviewed six randomized placebo-controlled trials (pharmacotherapy) of treatments for ataxia in MS. They concluded that there is insufficient information regarding absolute and comparative efficacy and tolerability of pharmacotherapies [70]. As a result, no recommendations could be given to guide in prescribing these medications [70].

It is worth mentioning that a patient-centered strategy is critical to the efficacy of pharmacological treatment, which is a crucial part of managing MS symptoms. To maximize compliance, particularly with invasive interventions, doctors must properly inform patients, discuss their priorities and expectations, and assist them in making the right treatment decisions [11]. With oral medications, the first dose should be low and gradually increased based on response and tolerability. If one medication is insufficient due to its ineffectiveness or unacceptable side effects, it is advised to combine several medications—possibly at lower doses [11].

6.2 Surgical interventions

Tremors can be both kinetic and postural, and they can be very challenging to manage. In case of tremor resistance to treatment, thalamotomy or thalamic stimulation has been tried to some degree of success [93]. Carefully selected patients with localized tremor with minimum disability could benefit from stereotactic thalamotomy, which targets the nucleus ventralis lateralis and nucleus ventralis intermedius, or DBS, which targets the nuclei ventralis lateralis and nucleus ventralis intermedius, ventralis oralis posterior nucleus, and zona incerta [94–96]. Tremor was abolished by both thalamotomy and thalamic stimulation in all patients immediately postsurgery [97]. However, tremor returned in almost all MS patients after 6 months, albeit of less severity than preoperative levels. Stereotactic thalamotomy seems to be more effective for intractable tremor, but the consequent functional improvement is variable and the intervention is associated with a higher risk of neurological deficit [11].

It is believed that distal tremor with good proximal stability and limb function are particularly responsive to DBS [11]. Successful alleviation of tremor in patients with MS has been achieved using DBS of the ventralis intermedius (VIM) thalamic nucleus [98]. Indeed, DBS is likely to improve tremor, but the effect might be reduced over time. Functional improvement is more often reported after DBS than after stereotactic thalamotomy, and DBS can be better tolerated. It has been reported that both procedures initially suppressed tremor in over 90% of patients, although functional improvement was seen only in 47.8% of those who underwent thalamotomy as opposed to 85.2% of those who had DBS [99]. However, the choice between interventions should be made on an individual basis in consultation with the specialist neurosurgical team [11], and larger trials that compare these two interventions and assess the efficacy are needed.

6.3 Rehabilitation approaches

Beyond pharmacological and surgical approaches, many physiotherapy approaches are used in balance therapy and tremor. Physiotherapy, orthoses, and limb cooling may be beneficial [20]. Indeed, in MS, rehabilitation programs may be helpful to enhance core stability in individuals with balance issues, lumbar stabilization exercises that strengthen the core trunk muscles and have an impact on postural control, ambulation, and skilled motor function [100]. A systemic review of trials with physical therapies showed some beneficial effect [101]. Additionally, Armutlu et al. [72] reported that physiotherapy approaches were effective to decrease the ataxia [7]. There is some evidence, according to a systematic review of research looking into the benefits of treadmill or robot-assisted training, that people with severe disabilities can see improvements in their quality of life and gait [102]. Two of the eight studies that were considered were modest single-group studies that only included individuals with progressing MS in their sample [103, 104]. Using weights and heavy walkers may decrease ataxic movements; however, they may increase fatigue [7, 105–107]. Patients with MS who were randomly assigned to physiotherapy showed improved scores on the Expanded Disability Status Scale (EDSS) and the Rivermead Mobility Index [7, 108]. An improvement in the Rivermead Mobility Index was seen in a different study on 42 randomly selected patients when home and outpatient therapy groups were compared to no therapy. However, mobility returned to pretreatment levels after 2 months of follow-up [109]. In MS patients, balance-based torso-weighting has been shown to improve cerebellar ataxia patients [110]. In 45 ataxic relapsing–remitting MS patients, the addition of core stability exercises and task-oriented training to typical balance training was found to potentially enhance stability [111]. Similar to this, task-oriented training and lumbar stabilization enhanced the efficacy of balance therapy in a group of 42 MS patients [74], exhibiting a considerable improvement in the International Cooperative Ataxia Rating Scale and composite balance scores. As measured by the International Cooperative Ataxia Rating Scale, the Mini-Balance Evaluation Systems Test, the smoothness of movement on both sides in a 5-m walk, and balance in a step-to-stand task before and after the intervention, a targeted ballet program aimed at reducing MS-associated ataxia and improving balance in women demonstrated significant clinical improvement [112]. These studies collectively demonstrate the positive effects of physiotherapy in MS-related ataxia [75]. In another study, it was determined that physiotherapy approaches were effective to decrease ataxia and that the combination of suitable physiotherapy techniques is effective in MS rehabilitation [7]. Even though physiotherapy has been shown to improve function in ataxia modestly, its long-term benefits in MS patients remain unclear.

Following task-specific rehabilitation, neural plasticity is enhanced [113, 114]. Thus, it is believed that balance and mobility interventions offer the proper task-specific stimuli to promote neural reorganization of central sensory integration, resulting in improved stability [6]. Despite the fact that neuroplasticity and motor learning are commonly considered to be more beneficial in the initial stages of MS, they seem to remain even in those with more severe disability [114]. Future research should establish whether or not those with progressive MS, and at different levels of disability, respond differently to these interventions, and if so whether and when interventions should be refocused on compensatory rather than restorative strategies.

DOI: http://dx.doi.org/10.5772/intechopen.112013

7. Conclusion

Ataxia is a common symptom of MS that can dramatically impact the patient's quality of life. The underlying pathophysiology of ataxia in MS is not fully understood, but it is believed to be related to demyelination and neurodegeneration in specific areas of the brain. There are currently no specific therapies approved for the treatment of ataxia in MS; however, several promising therapeutic approaches are being investigated, including the use of disease-modifying therapies, rehabilitative interventions, and symptomatic treatments.

8. Final remarks

This study demonstrates the complexity of understanding and targeting ataxia in MS. It provides a comprehensive overview of the most recent research and the current therapeutic strategies for managing ataxia in individuals with MS. It also highlights the multifactorial nature of the complex involvement of various brain regions, such as the cerebellum, brainstem, and spinal cord, in motor incoordination and impaired balance which might make their diagnosis and management difficult. There is still a lack of appropriate strategy in the treatment of ataxia in MS and in order to treat the complex character of ataxia, a multimodal strategy is urgently required. Finally, in order to better understand ataxia in MS and develop more effective treatments for this condition, ongoing research efforts and collaborative initiatives are of great importance.

Author details

Bilal El-Mansoury[1]*, Jawad Laadraoui[2], Abdelaati El Khiat[3,4], Omar El Hiba[1], Arumugam R. Jayakumar[5], Abdessalam Ferssiwi[1] and Abdelali Bitar[1]

1 Laboratory of Anthropogenic, Biotechnology and Health, Team Physiopathology Nutritional, Neurosciences and Toxicology, Faculty of Sciences, Chouaib Doukkali University, El Jadida, Morocco

2 Laboratory of Pharmacology, Neurobiology, Anthropology and Environment, Faculty of Sciences, Semlalia, Cadi Ayyad University, Marrakech, Morocco

3 Laboratory of Clinical and Experimental Neurosciences and Environment, Faculty of Medicine and Pharmacy, Cadi Ayyad University, Marrakech, Morocco

4 Biological and Health Sciences Team, Higher Institute of Nursing Professions and Health Techniques, Ministry of Health, Ouarzazate, Morocco

5 University of Miami School of Medicine, Miami, FL, USA

*Address all correspondence to: elmansoury1995bilal@gmail.com

References

[1] Dobson R, Giovannoni G. Multiple sclerosis–a review. European Journal of Neurology. 2019;**26**(1):27-40

[2] Frohman EM, Racke MK, Raine CS. Multiple sclerosis—The plaque and its pathogenesis. New England Journal of Medicine. 2006;**354**(9):942-955

[3] Wingerchuk DM, Lucchinetti CF, Noseworthy JH. Multiple sclerosis: Current pathophysiological concepts. Laboratory Investigation. 2001;**81**(3):263-281

[4] Maghzi A, Borazanci A, Mcgee J. 1 multiple sclerosis : Pathophysiology, clinical features, diagnosis, and management. In: Neuroinflammation. Amsterdam: Elsevier; 2011. DOI: 10.1016/B978-0-12-384913-7.00001-0

[5] Lublin FD, Reingold SC. Defining the clinical course of multiple sclerosis: Results of an international survey. Neurology. 1996;**46**(4):907-911

[6] Feinstein A, Freeman J, Lo AC. Progressive multiple sclerosis 2 treatment of progressive multiple sclerosis : What works, what does not , and what is needed. The Lancet Neurology. 2015;**14**(2):194-207. DOI: 10.1016/S1474-4422(14)70231-5

[7] Armutlu K, Karabudak R. Physiotherapy approaches in the treatment of ataxic multiple sclerosis : A pilot study. Neurorehabilitation and Neural Repair. 2001;**15**:203-211

[8] Correia de Sa JC, Airas L, Bartholome E, Grigoriadis N, Mattle H, Oreja-guevara C, et al. Symptomatic therapy in multiple sclerosis : A review for a multimodal approach in clinical practice. Therapeutic Advances in Neurological Disorders. 2011;**4**:139-168. DOI: 10.1177/1756285611403646

[9] Mills RJ, Yap L, Young CA. Treatment for ataxia in multiple sclerosis. Cochrane Database of Systematic Reviews. 2007;**1**:1-19

[10] Ben-zacharia AB, Ben-zacharia AB. Therapeutics for multiple sclerosis symptoms. Mount Sinai Journal of Medicine. 2011;**59**:176-191. DOI: 10.1002/MSJ

[11] Thompson AJ, Toosy AT, Ciccarelli O. Pharmacological management of symptoms in multiple sclerosis : Current approaches and future directions. The Lancet Neurology. 2010;**9**(12):1182-1199. DOI: 10.1016/S1474-4422(10)70249-0

[12] Petajan JH, White AT. Recommendations for physical activity in patients with multiple sclerosis. Sports Medicine. 1999;**27**(3):179-191

[13] Wilkins A. Cerebellar dysfunction in multiple sclerosis. Frontiers in Neurology. 2017;**8**(June):1-6. DOI: 10.3389/fneur.2017.00312

[14] Christensen H, Boysen G, Christensen AF, Johannesen HH. Insular lesions, ECG abnormalities, and outcome in acute stroke. Journal of Neurology, Neurosurgery & Psychiatry. 2005;**76**(2):269-271

[15] D'Ambrosio A, Pagani E, Riccitelli GC, Colombo B, Rodegher M, Falini A, et al. Cerebellar contribution to motor and cognitive performance in multiple sclerosis: An MRI sub-regional volumetric analysis. Multiple Sclerosis Journal. 2017;**23**(9):1194-1203

[16] Valentino P, Nisticò R, Pirritano D, Bilotti G, Del Giudice F, Sturniolo M, et al. Lamotrigine therapy for paroxysmal

dysarthria caused by multiple sclerosis: A case report. Journal of Neurology. 2011;**258**:1349-1350

[17] Weier K, Till C, Fonov V, Yeh EA, Arnold DL, Banwell B, et al. Contribution of the cerebellum to cognitive performance in children and adolescents with multiple sclerosis. Multiple Sclerosis Journal. 2016;**22**(5):599-607

[18] Kalincik T, Buzzard K, Jokubaitis V, Trojano M, Duquette P, Izquierdo G, et al. Risk of relapse phenotype recurrence in multiple sclerosis. Multiple Sclerosis Journal. 2014;**20**(11):1511-1522

[19] Ayache SS, Chalah MA, Al-ani T, Farhat WH, Zouari HG, Créange A, et al. Journal of the neurological sciences tremor in multiple sclerosis : The intriguing role of the cerebellum. Journal of the Neurological Sciences. 2015;**358**(1-2):351-356. DOI: 10.1016/j.jns.2015.09.360

[20] Koch M, Mostert J, Heersema D, De Keyser J. Tremor in multiple sclerosis. Journal of Neurology. 2007;**254**:133-145

[21] Alusi SH, Worthington J, Glickman S, Bain PG. A study of tremor in multiple sclerosis. Brain. 2001;**124**(4):720-730

[22] Pittock SJ, McClelland RL, Mayr WT, Rodriguez M, Matsumoto JY. Prevalence of tremor in multiple sclerosis and associated disability in the Olmsted County population. Movement Disorders. 2004;**19**(12):1482-1485

[23] Klockgether T. Ataxias: Diagnostic procedure and treatment. Der Nervenarzt. 2005;**76**:1275-1285

[24] Anheim M, Tranchant C, Koenig M. The autosomal recessive cerebellar ataxias. New England Journal of Medicine. 2012;**366**(7):636-646

[25] Durr A. Autosomal dominant cerebellar ataxias: Polyglutamine expansions and beyond. The Lancet Neurology. 2010;**9**(9):885-894

[26] Klockgether T. Acquired cerebellar ataxias and differential diagnosis. In: Blue Books of Neurology. Vol. 31. Amsterdam: Elsevier; 2007a. pp. 61-77

[27] Klockgether T. Update on degenerative ataxias. Current Opinion in Neurology. 2011;**24**(4):339-345

[28] Perlman SL. Spinocerebellar degenerations. Handbook of Clinical Neurology. 2011;**100**:113-140

[29] Teive HAG, Munhoz RP, Arruda WO, Raskin S, Werneck LC, Ashizawa T. Spinocerebellar ataxia type 10–a review. Parkinsonism & Related Disorders. 2011a;**17**(9):655-661

[30] Teive HAG, Munhoz RP, Ashizawa T. Inherited and sporadic ataxias. In: Hyperkinetic Movement Disorders: Differential Diagnosis and Treatment. Hoboken, New Jersey (United States): Wiley-Blackwell; 2011b. pp. 279-295

[31] Vermeer S, van de Warrenburg BPC, Willemsen M, Cluitmans M, Scheffer H, Kremer BP, et al. Autosomal recessive cerebellar ataxias: The current state of affairs. Journal of Medical Genetics. 2011;**48**(10):651-659

[32] Parisi MA. Clinical and molecular features of Joubert syndrome and related disorders. American Journal of Medical Genetics Part C: Seminars in Medical Genetics. 2009;**151**(4):326-340

[33] Romani M, Micalizzi A, Valente EM. Joubert syndrome: Congenital cerebellar ataxia with the molar tooth. The Lancet Neurology. 2013;**12**(9):894-905

[34] Shakkottai VG, Fogel BL. Clinical neurogenetics: autosomal dominant

spinocerebellar ataxia. Neurologic Clinics. 2013;**31**(4):987-1007

[35] Horvath R, Hudson G, Ferrari G, Fütterer N, Ahola S, Lamantea E, et al. Phenotypic spectrum associated with mutations of the mitochondrial polymerase γ gene. Brain. 2006;**129**(7):1674-1684

[36] Synofzik M, Srulijes K, Godau J, Berg D, Schöls L. Characterizing POLG ataxia: Clinics, electrophysiology and imaging. The Cerebellum. 2012;**11**:1002-1011

[37] Klockgether T. Sporadic adult-onset ataxia of unknown etiology. Handbook of Clinical Neurology. 2012;**103**:253-262

[38] Lin DJ, Hermann KL, Schmahmann JD. Multiple system atrophy of the cerebellar type: Clinical state of the art. Movement Disorders. 2014;**29**(3):294-304

[39] Van Gaalen J, Kerstens FG, Maas R, Härmark L, van de Warrenburg BPC. Drug-induced cerebellar ataxia: A systematic review. CNS Drugs. 2014;**28**:1139-1153

[40] Manto M. Toxic agents causing cerebellar ataxias. Handbook of Clinical Neurology. 2012;**103**:201-213

[41] Ariño H, Gresa-Arribas N, Blanco Y, Martínez-Hernández E, Sabater L, Petit-Pedrol M, et al. Cerebellar ataxia and glutamic acid decarboxylase antibodies: Immunologic profile and long-term effect of immunotherapy. JAMA Neurology. 2014;**71**(8):1009-1016

[42] Demarquay G, Honnorat J. Clinical presentation of immune-mediated cerebellar ataxia. Revue Neurologique. 2011;**167**(5):408-417

[43] Hadjivassiliou M, Aeschlimann P, Sanders DS, Mäki M, Kaukinen K, Grünewald RA, et al. Transglutaminase 6 antibodies in the diagnosis of gluten ataxia. Neurology. 2013;**80**(19):1740-1745

[44] Koeppen AH. Friedreich's ataxia: Pathology, pathogenesis, and molecular genetics. Journal of the Neurological Sciences. 2011;**303**(1-2):1-12

[45] Méneret A, Ahmar-Beaugendre Y, Rieunier G, Mahlaoui N, Gaymard B, Apartis E, et al. The pleiotropic movement disorders phenotype of adult ataxia-telangiectasia. Neurology. 2014;**83**(12):1087-1095

[46] Koeppen AH, Mazurkiewicz JE. Friedreich ataxia: Neuropathology revised. Journal of Neuropathology & Experimental Neurology. 2013;**72**(2):78-90

[47] Hou J-GG, Jankovic J. Movement disorders in Friedreich's ataxia. Journal of the Neurological Sciences. 2003;**206**(1):59-64

[48] Parkinson MH, Boesch S, Nachbauer W, Mariotti C, Giunti P. Clinical features of Friedreich's ataxia: Classical and atypical phenotypes. Journal of Neurochemistry. 2013;**126**:103-117

[49] Solbach K, Kraff O, Minnerop M, Beck A, Schöls L, Gizewski ER, et al. Cerebellar pathology in Friedreich's ataxia: Atrophied dentate nuclei with normal iron content. NeuroImage: Clinical. 2014;**6**:93-99

[50] Lynch DR, Perlman SL, Meier T. A phase 3, double-blind, placebo-controlled trial of idebenone in friedreich ataxia. Archives of Neurology. 2010;**67**(8):941-947

[51] Rinaldi C, Tucci T, Maione S, Giunta A, De Michele G, Filla A. Low-dose idebenone treatment in Friedreich's ataxia with and without cardiac hypertrophy. Journal of Neurology. 2009;**256**:1434-1437

[52] Pandolfo M, Arpa J, Delatycki MB, Le Quan Sang KH, Mariotti C, Munnich A, et al. Deferiprone in F riedreich ataxia: A 6-month randomized controlled trial. Annals of Neurology. 2014;**76**(4):509-521

[53] Soragni E, Miao W, Iudicello M, Jacoby D, De Mercanti S, Clerico M, et al. Epigenetic therapy for F riedreich ataxia. Annals of Neurology. 2014;**76**(4):489-508

[54] Verhagen MMM, Abdo WF, Willemsen M, Hogervorst FBL, Smeets D, Hiel JAP, et al. Clinical spectrum of ataxia-telangiectasia in adulthood. Neurology. 2009;**73**(6):430-437

[55] Hekman KE, Gomez CM. The autosomal dominant spinocerebellar ataxias: Emerging mechanistic themes suggest pervasive Purkinje cell vulnerability. Journal of Neurology, Neurosurgery & Psychiatry. 2015;**86**(5):554-561

[56] Matilla-DueñasA, AshizawaT, BriceA, Magri S, McFarland KN, Pandolfo M, et al. Consensus paper: Pathological mechanismsunderlyingneurodegeneration in spinocerebellar ataxias. The Cerebellum. 2014;**13**:269-302

[57] Rossi M, Perez-Lloret S, Doldan L, Cerquetti D, Balej J, Millar Vernetti P, et al. Autosomal dominant cerebellar ataxias: A systematic review of clinical features. European Journal of Neurology. 2014;**21**(4):607-615

[58] Balreira A, Boczonadi V, Barca E, Pyle A, Bansagi B, Appleton M, et al. ANO10 mutations cause ataxia and coenzyme Q 10 deficiency. Journal of Neurology. 2014;**261**:2192-2198

[59] Demos MK, van Karnebeek CDM, Ross CJD, Adam S, Shen Y, Zhan SH, et al. A novel recurrent mutation in ATP1A3 causes CAPOS syndrome. Orphanet Journal of Rare Diseases. 2014;**9**(1):1-9

[60] Heimdal K, Sanchez-Guixé M, Aukrust I, Bollerslev J, Bruland O, Jablonski GE, et al. STUB1 mutations in autosomal recessive ataxias–evidence for mutation-specific clinical heterogeneity. Orphanet Journal of Rare Diseases. 2014;**9**(1):1-12

[61] Liu Y-T, Hersheson J, Plagnol V, Fawcett K, Duberley KEC, Preza E, et al. Autosomal-recessive cerebellar ataxia caused by a novel ADCK3 mutation that elongates the protein: Clinical, genetic and biochemical characterisation. Journal of Neurology, Neurosurgery & Psychiatry. 2014;**85**(5):493-498

[62] Nanetti L, Cavalieri S, Pensato V, Erbetta A, Pareyson D, Panzeri M, et al. SETX mutations are a frequent genetic cause of juvenile and adult onset cerebellar ataxia with neuropathy and elevated serum alpha-fetoprotein. Orphanet Journal of Rare Diseases. 2013;**8**(1):1-9

[63] Renaud M, Anheim M, Kamsteeg E-J, Mallaret M, Mochel F, Vermeer S, et al. Autosomal recessive cerebellar ataxia type 3 due to ANO10 mutations: Delineation and genotype-phenotype correlation study. JAMA Neurology. 2014;**71**(10):1305-1310

[64] Synofzik M, Soehn AS, Gburek-Augustat J, Schicks J, Karle KN, Schüle R, et al. Autosomal recessive spastic ataxia of Charlevoix Saguenay (ARSACS): Expanding the genetic, clinical and imaging spectrum. Orphanet Journal of Rare Diseases. 2013;**8**(1):41

[65] Albanese A, Jankovic J. Hyperkinetic Movement Disorders: Differential Diagnosis and Treatment. Hoboken, New Jersey (United States): Wiley-Blackwell; 2012

[66] Klockgether T. Chapter 2 acquired cerebellar ataxias and differential diagnosis. In: Blue Books of Neurology. Vol. 31. Amsterdam: Elsevier; 2007b. DOI: 10.1016/S1877-184X(09)70076-0

[67] Teive HAG, Ashizawa T. Primary and secondary ataxias. Current Opinion in Neurology. 2015;**28**(4):413-422. DOI: 10.1097/WCO.0000000000000227

[68] Pérennou D, Thomas E-N, Blain H. Do French medical schools provide appropriate training on gait and gait disorders? Annals of Physical and Rehabilitation Medicine. 2011;**54**(1):36-47

[69] Ashizawa T, Xia G. Ataxia. Continuum: Lifelong Learning in Neurology. Movement Disorders. 2016;**22**(4):1208-1226

[70] Mills RJ, Yap L, Young CA. Treatment for ataxia in multiple sclerosis. Cochrane Database of Systematic Reviews. 2009;**1**:1-18

[71] Shah P. Symptomatic management in multiple sclerosis. Annals of Indian Academy of Neurology. 2015;**18**:35-42. DOI: 10.4103/0972-2327.164827

[72] Armutlu K, Karabudak R, Nurlu G. Physiotherapy approaches in the treatment of ataxic multiple sclerosis: A pilot study. Neurorehabilitation and Neural Repair. 2001;**15**(3):203-211

[73] Straudi S, Martinuzzi C, Pavarelli C, Sabbagh Charabati A, Benedetti MG, Foti C, et al. A task-oriented circuit training in multiple sclerosis: A feasibility study. BMC Neurology. 2014;**14**(1):1-9

[74] Salcı Y, Fil A, Armutlu K, Yildiz FG, Kurne A, Aksoy S, et al. Effects of different exercise modalities on ataxia in multiple sclerosis patients: A randomized controlled study. Disability and Rehabilitation. 2017;**39**(26):2626-2632

[75] Dubey S, Benito-león J. Movement disorders in multiple sclerosis : An update. Tremor Other Hyperkinet Mov (N Y). 2022;**12**(1):1-20. DOI: 10.5334/tohm.671

[76] Duquette P, Pleines J, du Souich P. Isoniazid for tremor in multiple sclerosis: A controlled trial. Neurology. 1985;**35**(12):1772

[77] Hallett M, Lindsey JW, Adelstein BD, Riley PO. Controlled trial of isoniazid therapy for severe postural cerebellar tremor in multiple sclerosis. Neurology. 1985;**35**(9):1374

[78] Koller WC. Pharmacologic trials in the treatment of cerebellar tremor. Archives of Neurology. 1984;**41**(3):280-281

[79] Schroeder A, Linker RA, Lukas C, Kraus PH, Gold R. Successful treatment of cerebellar ataxia and tremor in multiple sclerosis with topiramate: A case report. Clinical Neuropharmacology. 2010;**33**(6):317-318

[80] Sechi GP, Zuddas M, Piredda M, Agnetti V, Sau G, Piras ML, et al. Treatment of cerebellar tremors with carbamazepine: A controlled trial with long-term follow-up. Neurology. 1989;**39**(8):1113

[81] Feys P, D'hooghe MB, Nagels G, Helsen WF. The effect of levetiracetam on tremor severity and functionality in patients with multiple sclerosis. Multiple Sclerosis Journal. 2009;**15**(3):371-378

[82] Striano P, Coppola A, Vacca G, Zara F, Brescia Morra V, Orefice G, et al. Levetiracetam for cerebellar tremor in multiple sclerosis: An open-label pilot tolerability and efficacy study. Journal of Neurology. 2006;**253**:762-766

[83] Vahlberg B, Lindmark B, Zetterberg L, Hellström K, Cederholm T.

Body composition and physical function after progressive resistance and balance training among older adults after stroke: An exploratory randomized controlled trial. Disability and Rehabilitation. 2017;**39**(12):1207-1214

[84] Fox P, Bain PG, Glickman S, Carroll C, Zajicek J. The effect of cannabis on tremor in patients with multiple sclerosis. Neurology. 2004;**62**(7):1105-1109

[85] Monaca-Charley C, Stojkovic T, Duhamel A, De Seze J, Ferriby D, Vermersch P. Double-blind crossover study with dolasetron mesilate, a 5-HT 3 receptor antagonist in cerebellar syndrome secondary to multiple sclerosis. Journal of Neurology. 2003;**250**:1190-1194

[86] Wade DT, Makela P, Robson P, House H, Bateman C. Do cannabis-based medicinal extracts have general or specific effects on symptoms in multiple sclerosis? A double-blind, randomized, placebo-controlled study on 160 patients. Multiple Sclerosis Journal. 2004;**10**(4):434-441

[87] Zajicek J, Fox P, Sanders H, Wright D, Vickery J, Nunn A, et al. Cannabinoids for treatment of spasticity and other symptoms related to multiple sclerosis (CAMS study): Multicentre randomised placebo-controlled trial. The Lancet. 2003;**362**(9395):1517-1526

[88] Twomey JA, Espir ML. Paroxysmal symptoms as the first manifestations of multiple sclerosis. Journal of Neurology, Neurosurgery & Psychiatry. 1980;**43**(4):296-304

[89] Francis DA, Grundy D, Heron JR. The response to isoniazid of action tremor in multiple sclerosis and its assessment using polarised light goniometry. Journal of Neurology, Neurosurgery & Psychiatry. 1986;**49**(1):87-89

[90] Morrow J, McDowell H, Ritchie C, Patterson V. Isoniazid and action tremor in multiple sclerosis. Journal of Neurology, Neurosurgery, and Psychiatry. 1985;**48**(3):282

[91] Sabra AF, Hallett M, Sudarsky L, Mullally W. Treatment of action tremor in multiple sclerosis with isoniazid. Neurology. 1982;**32**(8):912

[92] Schniepp R, Jakl V, Wuehr M, Havla J, Kümpfel T, Dieterich M, et al. Treatment with 4-aminopyridine improves upper limb tremor of a patient with multiple sclerosis: A video case report. Multiple Sclerosis Journal. 2013;**19**(4):506-508

[93] Torres CV, Moro E, Lopez-Rios A-L, Hodaie M, Chen R, Laxton AW, et al. Deep brain stimulation of the ventral intermediate nucleus of the thalamus for tremor in patients with multiple sclerosis. Neurosurgery. 2010;**67**(3):646-651

[94] Bittar RG, Hyam J, Nandi D, Wang S, Liu X, Joint C, et al. Thalamotomy versus thalamic stimulation for multiple sclerosis tremor. Journal of Clinical Neuroscience. 2005;**12**(6):638-642

[95] Schuurman PR, Bosch DA, Bossuyt PMM, Bonsel GJ, Van Someren EJW, De Bie RMA, et al. A comparison of continuous thalamic stimulation and thalamotomy for suppression of severe tremor. New England Journal of Medicine. 2000;**342**(7):461-468

[96] Schuurman PR, Bosch DA, Merkus MP, Speelman JD. Long-term follow-up of thalamic stimulation versus thalamotomy for tremor suppression. Movement Disorders. 2008;**23**(8):1146-1153

[97] Zirh A, Reich SG, Dougherty PM, Lenz FA. Stereotactic thalamotomy in the treatment of essential tremor of the

upper extremity: Reassessment including a blinded measure of outcome. Journal of Neurology, Neurosurgery & Psychiatry. 1999;**66**(6):772-775

[98] Wishart HA, Roberts DW, Roth RM, McDonald BC, Coffey DJ, Mamourian AC, et al. Chronic deep brain stimulation for the treatment of tremor in multiple sclerosis: Review and case reports. Journal of Neurology, Neurosurgery & Psychiatry. 2003;**74**(10):1392-1397

[99] Yap L, Kouyialis A, Varma TRK. Stereotactic neurosurgery for disabling tremor in multiple sclerosis: Thalamotomy or deep brain stimulation? British Journal of Neurosurgery. 2007;**21**(4):349-354

[100] Freeman JA, Gear M, Pauli A, Cowan P, Finnigan C, Hunter H, et al. The effect of core stability training on balance and mobility in ambulant individuals with multiple sclerosis: A multi-Centre series of single case studies. Multiple Sclerosis Journal. 2010;**16**(11):1377-1384

[101] Fonteyn EMR, Keus SHJ, Verstappen CCP, Schöls L, de Groot IJM, van de Warrenburg BPC. The effectiveness of allied health care in patients with ataxia: A systematic review. Journal of Neurology. 2014;**261**:251-258

[102] Swinnen E, Beckwée D, Pinte D, Meeusen R, Baeyens J-P, Kerckhofs E. Treadmill training in multiple sclerosis: Can body weight support or robot assistance provide added value? A systematic review. Multiple Sclerosis International. 2012;**2012**:240274

[103] Giesser B, Beres-Jones J, Budovitch A, Herlihy E, Harkema S. Locomotor training using body weight support on a treadmill improves mobility in persons with multiple sclerosis: A pilot study. Multiple Sclerosis Journal. 2007;**13**(2):224-231

[104] Pilutti LA, Lelli DA, Paulseth JE, Crome M, Jiang S, Rathbone MP, et al. Effects of 12 weeks of supported treadmill training on functional ability and quality of life in progressive multiple sclerosis: A pilot study. Archives of Physical Medicine and Rehabilitation. 2011;**92**(1):31-36

[105] De Souza L. Multiple Sclerosis: Approaches to Management. Vol. 18. New York, NY: Springer; 2013

[106] Erickson HP, Lie MR, Wineinger MA. Rehabilitation in multiple sclerosis. Mayo Clinic Proceedings. 1989;**64**(7):818-828

[107] Morgan MH. Ataxia and weights. Physiotherapy. 1975;**61**(11):332-334

[108] Lord SE, Wade DT, Halligan PW. A comparison of two physiotherapy treatment approaches to improve walking in multiple sclerosis: A pilot randomized controlled study. Clinical Rehabilitation. 1998;**12**(6):477-486

[109] Wiles CM, Newcombe RG, Fuller KJ, Shaw S, Furnival-Doran J, Pickersgill TP, et al. Controlled randomised crossover trial of the effects of physiotherapy on mobility in chronic multiple sclerosis. Journal of Neurology, Neurosurgery & Psychiatry. 2001;**70**(2):174-179

[110] Widener GL, Conley N, Whiteford S, Gee J, Harrell A, Gibson-Horn C, et al. Changes in standing stability with balance-based torso-weighting with cerebellar ataxia: A pilot study. Physiotherapy Research International. 2020;**25**(1):e1814

[111] Ali AS, Darwish MH, Shalaby NM, Abbas RL, Soubhy HZ. Efficacy of core stability versus task oriented trainings on balance in ataxic persons with multiple sclerosis. A single blinded randomized controlled trial. Multiple Sclerosis and Related Disorders. 2021;**50**:102866

[112] Scheidler AM, Kinnett-Hopkins D, Learmonth YC, Motl R, López-Ortiz C. Targeted ballet program mitigates ataxia and improves balance in females with mild-to-moderate multiple sclerosis. PLoS One. 2018;**13**(10):e0205382

[113] Morgen K, Kadom N, Sawaki L, Tessitore A, Ohayon J, McFarland H, et al. Training-dependent plasticity in patients with multiple sclerosis. Brain. 2004;**127**(11):2506-2517

[114] Tomassini V, Johansen-Berg H, Leonardi L, Paixao L, Jbabdi S, Palace J, et al. Preservation of motor skill learning in patients with multiple sclerosis. Multiple Sclerosis Journal. 2011;**17**(1):103-115

Section 3

Interventions

Chapter 5

Adapted Physical Activity and Ataxia

Katerina Asonitou and Dimitra Koutsouki

Abstract

Ataxia affects the neurological system by impairing balance and motor coordination, which results in significant sensorimotor impairment in both children and adults. Physical activity (PA) has been linked to changes in the structure and functionality of the brain as well as effects on brain plasticity, according to numerous experimental and clinical studies. PA can help with concerns with standing and walking, fine and gross motor function regulation, and muscular tone. This chapter discusses the effects of various training programs on people with ataxia. Exercises that target balance, coordination, and muscular strength include: a) physical activity; b) treadmill training; c) locomotor training on a treadmill; d) trunk stabilization training; e) overground walking for balance; f) intensive exercises; and g) body-controlled videogames (exergames) played at home. Exercise and physical activity must be done frequently to maintain health, wellbeing, and quality of life. The duration and severity of the disease have an impact on how well adapted physical activity works.

Keywords: adapted physical activity, training exercises, ataxia, intervention, rehabilitation

1. Introduction

> *"Lack of activity destroys the good condition of every human being, while movement and methodical physical exercise save it and preserve it." – Plato (ancient Greek philosopher, 427–347 BCE).*

Inherited degenerative ataxia (DA) represents a clinically varied range of inheritance patterns, including autosomal dominant, autosomal recessive, X-linked, and mitochondrial. Hereditary ataxias with distinct mapped brain structures include fragile X tremor ataxia syndrome (FXTAS), ataxia telangiectasia (AT), ataxia with oculomotor apraxia types 1 and 2 (AOA1, AOA2), cerebellar ataxia/neuropathy/vestibular are flexia syndrome (CANVAS), and spinocerebellar ataxia (SCA). However, many inherited DA cases are idiopathic. A person's freedom and quality of life are negatively impacted by this group of disorders, which are characterized by a progressive deterioration in balance and coordination [1].

Cerebellar degeneration may result from inherited genetic mutations. Control over coordination is located in the cerebellum. The consequent lack of coordination in the lower and upper limbs, trunk, and neck affects all activities such as walking, standing, being on all fours, kneeling, squatting, sitting, controlling gestures, controlling speech, initiating an action, and stopping an action. Movements involving the fingers, hands, eyes, and voice are also affected. Because of this, the central nervous system's various regions and the communication pathways that carry information to them are dysfunctional, resulting in the typical ataxia symptoms [2].

There is currently no cure, and both medical and surgical interventions have only minor effects [2]. However, rehabilitative training regimens are advantageous for this population. By reducing the risk of the most prevalent age-related diseases, such as cardiovascular disease, stroke, diabetes, obesity, metabolic disorder, inflammation, muscle atrophy, bone and cartilage loss or degeneration, a decline in aerobic capacity, and the progression of several neurodegenerative diseases, physical activity has been shown in the literature to improve overall health. There is proof that living an active lifestyle and having good health go hand in hand [3–5] (**Figure 1**).

Exercise benefits all of the physiological systems in the human body, including the digestive, immune, circulatory, respiratory, and musculoskeletal systems [7]. Additionally, the benefits of exercise for brain health may slow the cognitive loss associated with aging. Regular exercise enhances cognition, memory, attention, processing speed, and executive function in healthy individuals and reduces the risk of dementia and other age-related cognitive illnesses [8, 9]. The authors recommend that future studies examine the amount of exercise that will best promote protection.

Exercise promotes pre- and postsynaptic function, synaptic plasticity, neurogenesis (neuroplasticity), and neuronal number [10]. Astrocytic degeneration, astrocyte size, and astrocyte levels may also increase [11] (**Figure 2**).

Maugeri and her colleagues conducted research on the effects of exercise on brain function in 2021, concentrating on the activity of astrocytes in a healthy central nervous system. They observed astrocytes and exercise have a positive relationship, and astrocyte changes may play a significant role in the improvement of executive and cognitive brain processes that is associated with exercise. The findings of this review showed the importance of exercise as a reliable and commonly used method

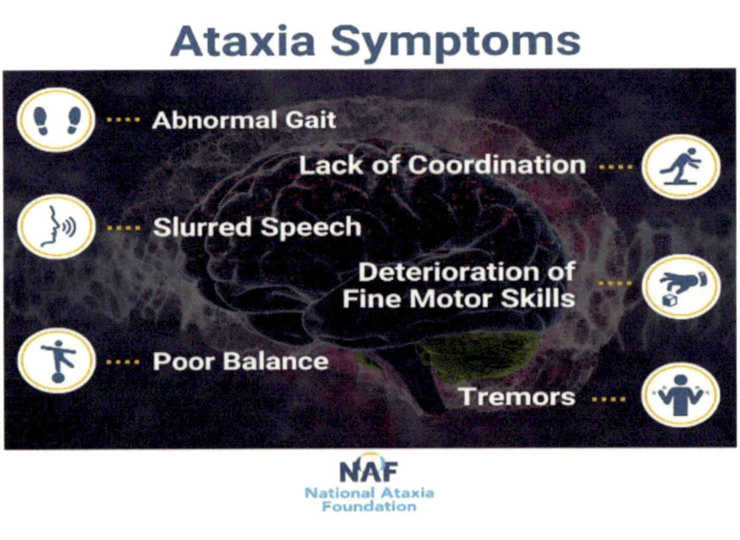

Figure 1.
Common ataxia symptoms [6].

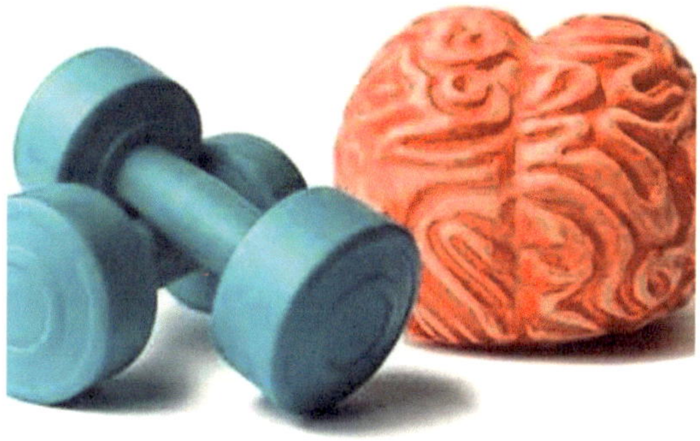

Figure 2.
Mental benefits of weight training [12].

for improving cognitive brain functioning through mechanisms that also include astrocytes. Even if it cannot be used alone, exercise is a potential treatment for neuropathologies [13].

There has been some research on the hippocampus, a vital brain area for memory and learning [14]. After participating in aerobic exercise for many months to a year, the prefrontal and temporal cortex [15], as well as the hippocampus [16], have all been shown to have increased activity and volume. In order to successfully support "brain rejuvenation" in important executive and cognitive domains, exercise is recommended.

2. Adapted physical activity

Structured group exercises are a part of adaptive physical activity (APA), which aims to improve patients' lifestyle, well-being, and quality of life [17]. Common phases are included in each training session: Warming up is followed by moderate-intensity aerobic activities, which are crucial for the harmonious stimulation of the entire body, strength exercises (such as a series of repetitions of 10 exercises for each muscle group), and exercises to increase venous return and energy restoration during cooling down. The APA program should include stretching activities for the stomach and upper/lower limb muscles, as well as limb mobility exercises for the head and shoulders.

Additionally, it uses basic, adaptable, light, and colorful equipment (such as elastics, sticks, hula hoops, bottles, balls, walls, rugs, and lesser weights for the barbell exercises) to enhance motor function, coordination, and motivation [18]. Additionally, the favorable effects of music on mood, motivation, and socializing during practice cannot be overstated. Particularly, SCA patients who consistently work out in the gym had improved psycho-physical health, which suggests reduced rates of anxiety and depression [19].

Due to its positive effects on neuromuscular rehabilitation of degenerative conditions such cerebellar ataxia, Parkinson's disease, and multiple sclerosis, dancing, and tai chi (a balance-based exercise) have gained popularity recently [1]. A case study by Song and his colleagues from 2019 had a patient with severe SCA who was 39 years old. They took part in an 8-week partnered tango dancing therapy program that was modified for intervention. His overall ataxia symptoms did not change, but his standing balance, gait, functional mobility, and quality of life did improve. Additionally, many of the improvements vanished one month after therapy [20].

The effects of 12 weeks of Tai Chi training on dynamic balance and disease severity were studied in 24 patients with cerebellar ataxia [21]. Twelve participants were randomly assigned to receive conventional treatment and twelve to participate in a tai chi intervention. Dynamic balance was assessed using the Berg Balance Scale (BBS), Scale for Assessment and Evaluation of Ataxia (SARA), SARAbal balance subcomponent, Sensory Organization Test, and Limits of Stability Test. Disease severity and health-related quality of life were assessed using the SARA and EuroQol visual analog scales, respectively. At baseline (week 0), after the intervention (week 12), and at the end of the 24-week follow-up period (week 36).

Three 60-minute sessions each week of the eight-part Tai Chi exercise program were part of the 12-week intervention. Participants were expected to perform tai chi at home alone for the ensuing 24 weeks. Although they participated in all programs, the control group received no help. The results showed that the experimental group's dynamic balance improved after 12 weeks of tai chi instruction. The increases, however, were not kept up during the 24-week follow-up evaluation period. Tai chi training did not lessen the severity of the problem, but after 12 weeks in this cohort, it did improve dynamic balance right away [21]. Tai chi and yoga have many similarities. People with cerebral palsy and ataxia can benefit from yoga by practicing it to relax their muscles and avoid atrophy.

The Duret et al. study [22] examined the outcomes of a 6-month modified physical activity-based program (APA-program) designed for patients who reside in their communities (mean age 59 14 years) and had experienced 47 strokes, 13 episodes of multiple sclerosis, and 19 other neurological illnesses. This APA program included both individual and group workouts, and it was led by an APA instructor twice a week in local fitness centers. The six-minute walk test (6MWT), the single-leg stance test (SLST), and the Short Form-36 (SF-36) were all strength tests carried out on exercise equipment. Standing time on one leg increased by 86%, standing time on one leg grew by 22%, upper body strength increased by 49%, lower body strength increased by 37%, and SF-36 Mental and Physical scores increased by 23%.

The quality of life and all physical capacities both increased.

At the end of the six-month program, more than half of participants (83%) decided to buy a one-year gym membership, enabling the development of community APA-programs for persons with chronic neurological disorders in collaboration with rehabilitation institutions. 68 percent of participants finished the course. The conclusion of this research paper's most important section contains the author's conclusions and recommendations: A program based on physical activity delivered in a gym effectively improves the physical health and quality of life for people with neurological conditions like multiple sclerosis and stroke; b) collaboration between rehabilitation clinics and nearby fitness centers, instruction in adapted physical activity from qualified instructors, and group activities are crucial elements for successful participation [22].

2.1 Physical exercises based on coordination, balance, and muscular strength

He and co-workers [1] conducted a systematic review through five electronic databases (Cochrane Library, Physiotherapy Evidence Database (PEDro), EMbase, PubMed and MEDLINE) including articles from 1999 to 2020 concerning the effectiveness of balance and coordination training in patients with inherited degenerative ataxia. A total of 515 publications were initially retrieved but only 33 of them met the eligibility criteria. They were categorized by their interventions and study design. Three rehabilitation methods were examined: a) conventional physical/occupational therapy, b) virtual reality/videogame-based training, and c) adapted physical activity.

The results showed that static/dynamic balance and coordination training as a intervened tool in the field of the conventional physical/occupational therapy can improve more effectively the balance and coordinative function of patients with genetic DA. Current literature has shown that this rehabilitation method improve gait, motor function and other ataxia symptoms without causing major adverse effects. Leg cycling and core stability training have also been reported as effective tools in improving dynamic balance in progressive degenerative cerebellar ataxia. The use of proprioceptive stabilizer, vibration assisted therapy, and neuromodulation facilitates motor learning enhancing the effect of conventional physical therapy on DA [1].

Strength training and dynamic postural balance can improve motor coordination of limbs and trunks giving to patients a better lifestyle either walking or in a wheelchair. The effectiveness of a more functional gait as well sitting and standing without help was observed in a 24-week intervention study [23] as well a case study [24]. In the 24-week intervention study participated 38 spinocerebellar ataxia type patients who received 6 hours of neurorehabilitation therapy, emphasizing on balance, coordination, and muscle strengthening on weekdays. In the case study 3 male patients 20–30-year received 45 min—1 h per session, daily for 12 weeks, 3 days in supervision of therapists and remaining days at home. The constant benefits through strength training were the regression of ataxia symptoms, such as limb tremors and imbalances. After training, patients gained more mobility controlled and functional independence [23, 24].

Salci and colleagues investigated the effects of different exercise protocols for 42 ataxia patients with multiple sclerosis. Participants were divided into three different groups: a balance training (BT) group, a lumbar stabilization (LS) group and a task-oriented training (TT) group. Within 18 training sessions all these groups received balance training. The LS group also received specific lumbar stabilization exercises. The TT group received task-oriented training. The results showed significant improvements; however, balance training alone is not enough for the rehabilitation of these patients. A combination of lumbar stabilization exercises or task-oriented training enhance the benefits of balance rehabilitation [25].

2.2 Treadmill training and overground walking for balance and gait

According to a case report by Cernak and associates published in 2008, a 13-year-old girl with severe cerebellar ataxia who was not mobile improved in walking ability with a treadmill training program. Her long-term goal was to be able to independently move around her house with a walker. The intervention strategy involves both floor-based walking and treadmill exercise training using a body weight support system (BWS). It was done at a clinic five days a week for four weeks. Five days a week, for 20 minutes per session, exercise training with the BWS was continued for four months at home. The results showed an improvement in stride length and velocity. Exercise training utilizing BWS on a treadmill combined with ground-based gait training may be a useful approach to improve walking abilities in those with severe cerebellar ataxia. The amount and duration of training, however, can be increased to achieve functionally meaningful gains [26].

A comparable longitudinal case study with a specialist personal trainer was carried out in a gym [27]. An exercise program was completed by a 43-year-old man with motor ataxia, and his performance was evaluated both before and after the test. For six months, there were two 30-minute training sessions per week that targeted body stabilization, strength, and cardiovascular fitness. One month later, the post-test was completed. The following seven things were rated using the Scale for the Assessment and Rating of Ataxia (SARA): 1. Gait 2. Position 3. seated. 4. Finger Snatching. 5. The nasal finger test. 6. Quick hand motions that alternate. 7. Heel-chin slide. Additionally, balance exercises for standing and sitting were included of the rehabilitation regimen.

The clinical scale for the Assessment and Rating of Ataxia (SARA) is most typically used to assess a variety of distinct cerebellar ataxia abnormalities, including Friedreich's ataxia, ataxic stroke, and spinocerebellar ataxia. Reliability and validity were initially published in 2006, were certified [28], and were extensively used to assess the severity and development of disease in clinical practice and longitudinal investigations [1–3].

Exercises of varying degrees of difficulty were performed during the training sessions, including back rowing (3x: 8,10,12 repetitions), chest and shoulder presses (3x: 8,10,12 repetitions), assisted walking on the treadmill (15 m), spinning on the bike (15 m), astatic body stabilization (2x: 1 m), glute stabilization (2x: 15 repetitions), leg presses (3x: 8,10,12 repetitions), leg extensions (3x: 8,10,12 repetitions), elliptical training (3x: 10,15,20 repetitions), trunk lift on inclined platform and with medicine ball (2x: 15 repetitions), front swing with kettlebell (3x: 8,10,12 repetitions), butterfly (3x: 8,10,12 repetitions), reverse butterfly (3x: 8,10,12 repetitions), squat with and without load (3x: 8,10,12 repetitions to 12, 15, 20 repetitions depending on load), rope jumping (5x: 30s), hill climbing on elliptical trainer (2x: 30s), Jumping jacks (5 times for 30 counts), deadlifts with parallel bars (3 times for 10, 15, and 20 repetitions), TRX rows (3 times for 10, 15, and 20 repetitions), Russian twists with medicine balls (2 times for 30 counts), hack squats (3 times for 10, 15, and 20 counts), push-ups with hands (3 times for 10, 15, and 20 counts), wall ball and lunges with disks on the head (3 times for 20, 25, and 30 reps). A variety of exercises were used, depending on the goal of each session [27]. The treadmill itself might be a useful instrument. This program may enhance the health, happiness, and quality of life for people with ataxia. The findings showed improvements in blood pressure and body composition, as well as gains in all SARA scale items except than "sitting" and "finger chase," where the value remained same [27].

Similar studies [26, 29] demonstrated that patients with cerebellar syndrome benefit from three times per week of treadmill exercise for improving gait parameter. Less gait assistance was needed after the training program, and the walking distance had increased. The usage of these activities, according to the authors, is advised for people who are no longer able to walk. Additionally, it has been shown that patients' quality of life can be improved by greater mobility in later stages of cerebellar degeneration [30, 31]. This study [27] also established the proper level of intervention. Because rehabilitation cannot stop the progression of cerebellar degeneration, this is a significant contribution to the research. In summary, this study offers support for the use of physical exercise regimens in ataxia patients.

Previous studies concluded that patients with SCA can benefit long-term from motor activity and physical exercise if they engage in steady and continuous motor activity. However, the clinical effect is quickly lost once this activity is terminated [32]. Future longitudinal training studies should therefore monitor this problem and maximize functioning throughout.

2.3 Locomotor training using a treadmill/intensive exercises

A systematic review study conducted by Milne and colleagues examined 7 categories of intervention for individuals with genetic degenerative ataxia: a) coordination and balance training, b) multifaceted inpatient rehabilitation, c) a cycling regime, d) balance training (exercises with technology assisted biofeedback), e) treadmill training, f) occupational therapy, and g) respiratory muscle training. Seventeen (17) studies met the criteria for long-term outcomes, optimal duration, and intensity of rehabilitation and included in this review [33].

The results highlighted the different types of intervention regarding intensity and duration. Preliminary findings suggested that multifaceted programs incorporating more than one type of intervention, such as coordination and balance training, may have greater effect than isolated rehabilitation programs, such as only balance training or occupational therapy. Significant within-group outcomes suggested that improvements in balance can occur at 3 weeks, and improvements in ataxia require a minimum of 4 weeks.

Intensity as the duration of intervention programs appears to have similar effectiveness. Subgroup analyses indicate improved effectiveness with greater rehabilitation intensity; 60 minutes or greater for 2 days or more per week appears more effective than less intensive training program. The results were less clear for functional gains regarding the duration and benefits beyond 3 days [33].

A crucial new piece of knowledge came from the Miyai et al. study, which examined the short- and long-term effects of intensive rehabilitation on gait and activities of daily living (ADLs) in people with progressive cerebellar ataxia. There was a total of 42 patients in the immediate group and the control group. The immediate group received physical and occupational therapy for two hours on weekdays and one hour on weekends for a period of four weeks, with a focus on balance, coordination, and ADLs. The control group received the same therapy but with a 4-week delay. The results showed that patients with degenerative ataxia benefit from and tolerate a 2-hour daily program well. Short-term outcomes between the two groups were examined. The highest level of rehabilitation intensity gave the largest advantages, which sustained in more than half of the participants, even though the functional status of participants tended to revert to baseline within 24 weeks [34]. Patients in both groups had long-term follow-up data collected up to 24 weeks after the intervention. Each outcome measure for the long-term result was evaluated prior to (pre) and immediately following (post) the intervention for 4 weeks as well as at 4 weeks, 12 weeks, and 24 weeks passed in both groups after the intervention.

Long-term follow-up showed that, as we predicted, the improvements ultimately diminished. Ilg and colleagues {24} found that patients with cerebellar ataxia but not those with afferent ataxia benefited from a less frequent intervention of one hour of physical therapy administered three times weekly for four weeks. With a self-directed home workout regimen, the impact persisted for 8 weeks. Their view is consistent with our findings that improvements in gait speed and SARA persisted for 12 and 24 weeks, respectively. We demonstrated that the SARA score decreased to baseline at 24 weeks in addition to their findings. There are at least two reasons that could account for this drop. Cerebellar lesions may affect the first consolidation of the encoded motor skill. Second, the advancing degenerative process itself might impair motor function. After an intense intervention, systemic self-exercise and intermittent home therapy may be required to maintain functional status [34].

Although frequent rehabilitation programs focusing on balance, walking, and ADLs may lessen impairment and its associated handicap despite significant cerebellar damage, such motor learning depends on both the cerebellum and basal ganglia systems. Ataxia did demonstrate improvement in the trunk, but it also significantly improved in the limbs. This suggests that the effect cannot be fully explained by the encouragement of physical fitness. Patients with cerebellar injury have poorer motor learning, according to earlier investigations. Most of the research, however, employed a stimulus-response methodology, suggesting that action-based working memory, rather than a learning mechanism, may have an impact on performance. In fact, when the replies were given a direct cue, patients with cerebellar degeneration displayed improved sequence learning.

Although fewer falls could be a desirable outcome in daily living, the intervention did not lower risk for falls. Environmental factors and practice at home may be more significant than therapy in a hospital. Finally, the study's examination of patient subgroups showed that patients with mild ataxia benefited the most from rigorous rehabilitation. It is necessary to investigate an optimal intervention for those with moderate to severe ataxia. Further research will be required to determine whether a multimodal strategy involving neuromodulation, rehabilitation, brain stimulation, and neuropharmacological therapy, such as thyrotropin-releasing hormone, may improve functional result. In conclusion, it is proposed that patients with degenerative cerebellar illnesses can at least partially overcome reduced motor learning by intensive and concentrated rehabilitation. Additional research will be required to establish the ideal dosage, durations, and spacing between therapies to maintain substantial functional improvements [34].

The longitudinal case study by Honorio et al. might lend support to earlier case studies that advocated for frequent and intense training [27]. Additionally, Milne et al.'s systematic review study validates and supports that exercise therapies such as coordination and balance training, balance exercises, respiratory muscle training, and treadmill training can improve the participants' quality of life [33].

2.4 Trunk stabilization training-postural exercises- trunk muscle performance

Postural instability is a basic clinical feature of SCA related to static, and dynamic imbalance, difficulties in gait and mobility, fallings with a risk of bone fractures and other complications. These outcomes often lead to refusal of physical activity and consequent social isolation. SCA-related rigidity is a main cause of postural instability and is associated with postural destabilizing and other abnormal reactions. Treatment strategies should consider podalic and visual receptor stimulation. Structural exercises are implemented to improve muscular strength and balance using fitball as a wall squat, single wall squat, balance reversal lunge, balance push-up, ball pass, and balance oblique crunch [18].

Moreover, in some cases postural instability may lead to chronic lumbar backache. Stretching of lumbar muscles by using specific methods, such as Pilates, Mezieres, and Feeldenkrais is an important rehabilitation exercise (**Figure 3**).

On the other hand, physical activities of daily living (e.g., getting up from a chair, holding and throwing objects, and the standing position) in conjunction with "re-learning" of destabilizing responses (e.g., by using moving platforms) are essential components of interventional approach [18].

The motor activity program in the fields of adapted physical activity, kinesitherapy, and physiotherapy includes the preparatory and operational phase. The first aims

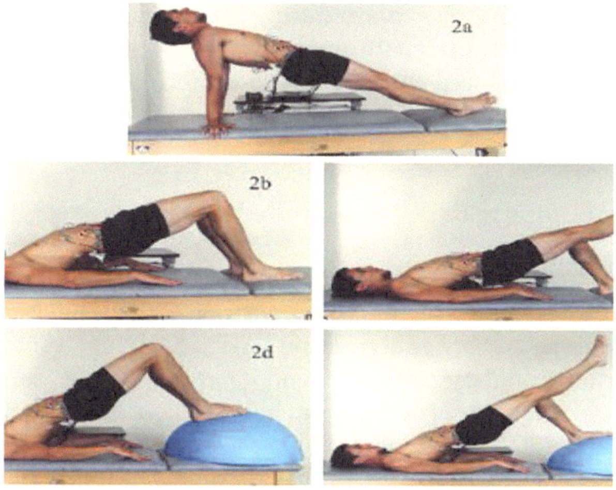

Figure 3.
Trunk stabilization exercises: a) elbows extended; b) conventional back-bridge; c) elevated right leg; d) feet resting on the BOSUTM balance trainer; e) left foot on BOSUTM balance trainer and elevated right leg [35].

to learn the patient's own body perception, spatial-time awareness, coordination, respiration, and simple motor movements. The second, progressively learns complex tasks, by repetition of the activities, with result to enhance patients' sensorial experience, executive strategies, and anticipatory capabilities [36].

Due to limited diagnostic methods and scientific evidence in the last years researchers have focused on different rehabilitative techniques. The motor recovery and adaptation after the cerebellar degeneration involves synaptic plasticity. So the intervention programs of motor dysfunction have mostly focused on exercises of balance, stretching, coordination, proprioception, and walking [18].

Also, trunk weighting has been recommended for postural and movement control with reduction of coordination disorders and improvement of balance and gait [26–29]. A treatment that includes the addition of small weights on the torso is a promising intervention that may improve balance and mobility.

The scientific feasibility of BBTW (balance-based torso-weighting) for improving standing stability proved in patients with multiple sclerosis as well ataxia [37]. In this single-session quasi-experimental pilot study participated 10 individuals with cerebellar ataxia and 10 matched controls. For standing stability was used the modified Clinical Test of Sensory Interaction on Balance mCTSIB; [38]. All participants stood for up to 30secods (or for shorter time if the person moved their feet out of position or needed assistance to prevent falling) on firm and foam surfaces with eyes open then eyes closed for standing stability. For dynamic balance participants performed the Timed Up and Go test TUG; [39] where they stood up from a chair, walked 3 m, turned around, walked back, and sat down in the chair again. Light weights (0.57–1.25 kg) were strategically applied to a vestlike garment. The participants performed all testing tasks without weights before undergoing the BBTW procedure. After receiving BBTW weights, participants repeated the standing stability and TUG tasks [37].

Weighting training may be particularly useful in increasing stability of people with ataxia. However, functional movement speed did not improve. Additional variables such as testing accuracy (e.g., step length, step width, and percent of gait cycle in single- and double-limb support during gait) should be examined in the future research. Also, individuals with ataxia may use slower movement as a strategy to perform tasks, with the speed–accuracy trade-off formalized by Fitts' law [40]. Future studies should further examine gait stability measures along with movement speed [37].

2.5 Home-based training with body-controlled exergames

The body continuously adapts its motor and cognitive behavior when the senses are stimulated. The developing technology of virtual reality is being used to rehabilitative settings. Different activities in real time, such as playing, walking, and manipulating objects permit stimulation of senses and interactively operate. Indeed, this method can non-invasively improve motion, balance, coordination, and cognition.

Ten kids with mild SCA who could walk on their own participated in a study with three popular video game platforms. The 2-week study methodology focused on certain whole-body motions that can increase stability and reduce falls. Results from the post-treatment phase revealed improvement in SARA items pertaining to posture, balance, walking, and coordination. Although it is uncertain whether this method can be used with severe patients, the authors found that playing video games improves eye-motor coordination, anticipatory skills, and rapid motions to be conducted in a virtual world [41].

A similar exploratory study looked at SCA patients who were treated with a variety of videogames for 12 weeks while in a wheelchair. The findings indicated progress at SARA, but the authors recommended additional research to corroborate these preliminary findings [42]. at terms of the genre, coordination sports like table tennis, squash, badminton, and games of boules are advised at the beginning. To significantly enhance posture and coordination, perform these games on an elastic carpet [43].

To minimize falls and enhance mobility, resistance, posture, balance, and muscle strength in people with severe ataxia, video games or virtual reality therapy should be used in conjunction with a particular training regimen. Console games like Ski Slalom and Tightrope Walk offer exercises for both static and dynamic balance as well as whole-body movements (**Figure 4**).

3. Individualized education program and physical activity coaching intervention

Since fitness is a main goal of physical activity, Physical Education (PE) teachers or coaches should take in to account that individuals with disabilities generally display the same physiological responses to exercise found in non-disabled people. "Although specific disabilities may affect the intensity, duration, and frequency of exercise, individuals with disabilities can benefit from training improving their performances. Wheelchairs can be adjusted or modified (by those qualified to do so) to improve physical activity performance. Those practicing physical activities or athletes in wheelchairs play basketball, tennis, and many other sports" [45].

The Individual Education Program (IEP) is the basic tool of PE teachers who firstly evaluate the cognitive-motor profile of those practicing physical activities. Subsequently the instructor designs the IEP which focuses on short- and long-term goals and objectives for training of the patient. Individuals with disabilities (children and adolescents) are entitled to receive special services based on their

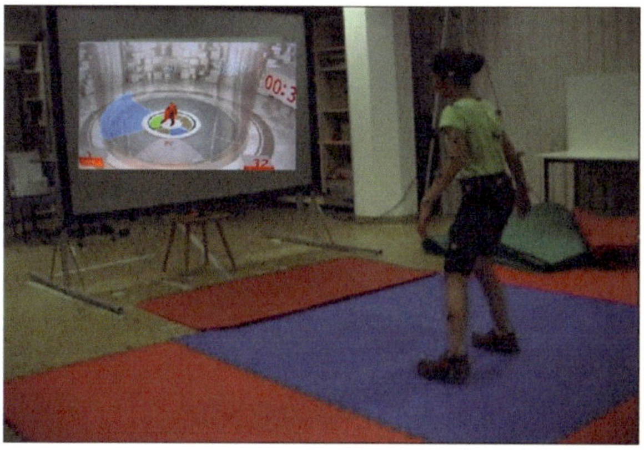

Figure 4.
Exergame-based training (e.g., Kinect games: a. 20.000 leaks trains whole-body coordination and engagement with a dynamic environment; b. table tennis trains goal-directed upper limb movements, dynamic balance, and movement timing; c. light racing trains goal-directed lower limb motions, quick movements, and dynamic balance) [44].

individual needs, which are determined by their assessment and evaluation. In a corresponding context Physical Activity Coaching Intervention is an Individualized Intervention Program (IIP) that take in to account the fitness profile and the individual characteristics of the patients to implement, for instance, a strength training program.

The PE instructor or coach should put the individual, not the disability, at the center of their planning when deciding how to instruct or train a student with a handicap. For instance, the instructor encourages the patient to continue attempting to build physical activity and health-related fitness with the goal of inclusion, challenges his intellect, and helps the patient stay on task longer. When working on basketball shooting techniques, for instance, the PE teacher or coach may also utilize modifications as a fundamental technique to make sure the patient feels competent and actively participates in the task. Given that he has trouble moving, you may try to make the basketball hoop smaller, use a lighter ball, or construct a basket that is worth more points.

Planned adaptations for physical activities include a modified setting, adjustments to the rules, the goal and content of the activities, and the rate of learning. For example, because field sports like baseball and soccer require adaptations, the surroundings will need to be changed when walkers and wheelchairs are used. Wheelchairs and walkers can also benefit from adaptive equipment, such as smaller or lower targets, areas on the playing field marked with cones, scoops for catching, and different balls (size, weight, color, and texture). "A person with cerebral palsy can stand up straight with the help of walkers or standing frames. The tool is helpful in maintaining range of motion, boosting endurance, and strengthening trunk muscles for cerebral palsy patients [45].

The term "least restrictive environment" refers to the practice of including people with disabilities as much as is practical in circumstances where their counterparts without impairments are present. "Empowerment is generally defined as a process through which individuals gain control over their lives, a sense of power equitable with others, and a feeling of responsibility for self, other, and environment" [46] (**Figure** 5).

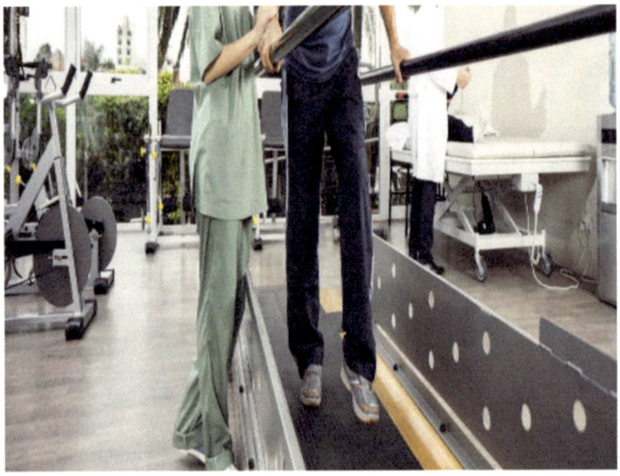

Figure 5.
Balance & Gait Disorders [47].

These two ideas are crucial for modification or adaptation in a learning environment when a PE instructor or coach wants to provide patients with ataxia with the least restrictive environment possible.

Maintaining one's health, wellbeing, and quality of life requires regular physical activity. The World Health Organization WHO, [48] suggests engaging in low to moderate intensity physical or recreational activities at least three times per week for a total of roughly 30 minutes per day. This can involve resistance training, aerobic exercise, or a combination of the two [48]. Regular aerobic training, manual wheelchair propulsion, arm cranking, swimming, and circuit training have all been shown to increase the cardiorespiratory fitness, upper extremity muscle strength, and endurance of wheelchair users. The patient's cardiometabolic profile is improved by aerobic exercise because it increases maximal oxygen consumption, improves cardiorespiratory status, and lowers blood glucose, body fat, and BMI levels. Patients also tend to engage in daily activities like wheelchair use, personal grooming, and cleaning their surroundings frequently [49].

For those who have neurodegenerative disorders, physical activity (PA) might be a potent neuroprotective intervention; unfortunately, rehabilitation programs frequently overlook methods to boost PA engagement. It has been demonstrated that the *Engage intervention* increases exercise self-efficacy and PA uptake in adults with ataxia, Parkinson's disease, and Huntington's disease. An ongoing single-cohort study called *Engage-Ataxia* is being conducted at Columbia University.

Over the course of 12 weeks, a physical therapist offered a 5-session coaching program (PA) via telemedicine. Based on the self-determination theory, the intervention featured a disease-specific workbook to direct the sessions and take into account balance and gait issues, deficiencies in motor learning, and weariness. Individualized workout advice, goal-setting, and strategies for overcoming movement challenges were all covered in the sessions. Only 19 of the 25 participants (mean age 55.8 years; SD: 13.7) completed the intervention (8 men; 11 women). To keep an eye on PA and heart rate, they used a Fitbit. The authors concluded that *Engage-Ataxia* offered a workable framework to increase PA in ataxia patients. This intervention was supported by preliminary results, which showed improvements in behavior change and disease-specific motor and cognitive function tests [50].

The practical benefit of evaluating ataxia patients for a variety of challenges and intensity, regardless of a specific medical diagnosis, is that a PE teacher can get a personalized appraisal of the patient's strengths and weaknesses. Future studies in program evaluation and design may be required to concentrate on patient profiles across a variety of domains (motor, cognitive, social, and emotional), examining each individual's strengths and limitations. Therefore, regardless of the diagnosis a patient receives, PE teachers and coaches will be able to modify their support in accordance and implement an effective IEP and IIP.

4. Final remarks and recommendation

Although supportive care is necessary to manage the symptoms, there is currently no treatment to halt the disease's progression. Issues with balance, poor voluntary movement coordination, double vision, slurred speech, and difficulties swallowing are among of the condition's most prevalent symptoms. Individuals may also experience stiffness and a loss of sensation resembling Parkinson's or multiple sclerosis.

A variety of rehabilitation programs may be helpful for ataxia patients. Physiotherapy can preserve muscle tone, improve strength and mobility overall, and stop joints from dislocating. Patients who need assistance utilizing adaptive equipment like a wheelchair, cane, or walker can benefit from occupational therapy. Speech and language therapy can help with swallowing and speech improvement. Other forms of therapy and treatment can include medical or pharmaceutical, healthy eating, getting enough sleep, conducting education, biofeedback, yoga, and surgery, among others. Adaptive physical activity, occupational therapy, and physical therapy are three professions that have a lot in common. They often practice the same abilities and clearly understand the importance of the underlying neuromuscular systems that regulate how motions are performed.

The APA intervention is described as a rehabilitation program as opposed to "therapy." Most rehabilitation methods are derived from basic physical activities like aerobic, muscle- and bone-strengthening, balancing, and flexibility exercises. Basic elements of physical activity are included even while utilizing exercise equipment, such as a treadmill, which is an aerobic/cardiovascular workout. People with severe ataxia may benefit from overground walking, trunk stabilization exercises, functional manipulative skills, sports, and leisure activities to help them improve their balance, gait, function, motor coordination, trunk, and movement performance.

The outcomes of an intervention training program are significantly influenced by its length. Adults with severe ataxia may benefit from a 6-month planned physical activity and focused training program since it will improve their general health by boosting their fitness levels, balance, and strength. Ataxia patients may become more involved in community outdoor activities, which will help them integrate with people who do not have disabilities, increase their physical fitness so they can manage daily tasks more easily, and adopt a happier, healthier lifestyle.

Susruta, Hippocrates, and Galen's contributions to the notion that *"exercise is medicine"*, along with the concept's historical context, show that the foundations for the exercise prescription for health and disease prevention has roots that go back more than two millennia in antiquity. Exercise and medical experts should be aware that Susruta, an Indus Valley physician who lived more than 2.5 millennia ago, was the first person to prescribe moderate daily exercise for this reason. They should also be aware that the first "recorded" physician to recommend writing exercise for a patient with a disease (consumption) was Hippocrates of Greece. He is widely regarded as the "father of medicine". Last but not least, Galen's influence led to the promotion of exercise for health benefits and to lessen the consequences of disease. Up until the beginning of the 16th century, he used exercise to cure patients suffering from a range of maladies [51]. However, current studies with a strong evidence-based data also indicate the advantages of physical activity for both physical and mental health [52, 53].

According to the results of other studies, adapted physical exercise and ataxia are associated with positive health outcomes that support an active lifestyle. The use of personalized physical activity-specific therapies to a larger sample of children, adolescents, and adults is also required, while taking sociocultural, gender, and age factors into consideration. Research is still needed to determine the number and length of treatments required to provide a higher chance of improvement and a higher chance that changes will last. Long-term research examining the best physical activity therapies for children and adolescents with different genetic ataxias are lacking.

Future research will be needed to maintain the advantages, determine the frequency that is most effective, as well as the dosage and delivery method. Ataxia patients can benefit from any sort or amount of intervention, according to this review of the domain of interventions. Due to the complexity of the disease and the unique characteristics, it is required to provide particular diagnoses, symptoms, or "severity" while conducting research in this population. This is significant because, while an intervention might be helpful for a population with ataxia that shares the same features (for example, speech issues), it might not be helpful without modifications for other individuals who have other characteristics (for example, issues other than speech issues).

The findings of this evaluation of the available literature support the necessity for further research into the efficacy of APA treatments for children and adolescents with generative ataxia. In order to better understand the effectiveness and safety of treatments for degenerative ataxia, longitudinal studies are also necessary in this field of research. And finally, the multidisciplinary team is always undeniably important in diagnosing and treating patients with ataxia. Ataxia patients typically receive reviews many times a year, ideally from a specialized team that comprises a neurologist, an advanced palliative care nurse, and, as necessary, additional medical professionals like psychiatrists, physiatrists, social workers, and others.

Adaptive physical activity intervention, occupational therapy, physiotherapy, speech and language therapy (for both feeding and communication), and other interventions can all be very helpful at different periods in the patient's life.

DOI: http://dx.doi.org/10.5772/intechopen.111792

Author details

Katerina Asonitou* and Dimitra Koutsouki
Laboratory of Adapted Physical Activity/Developmental and Physical Disabilities, School of Physical Education and Sport Science, National and Kapodistrian University of Athens, Athens, Greece

*Address all correspondence to: kasonitou@phed.uoa.gr

References

[1] He M, Zhang HN, Tang ZC, Gao SG. Balance and coordination training for patients with genetic degenerative ataxia: A systematic review. Journal of Neurology. 2021;**268**(10):3690-3705. DOI: 10.1007/s00415-020-09938-6

[2] Matsugi A. Physical therapy for cerebellar ataxia. In: Suzuuki T, editor. Neurological Physical Therapy 157. London, UKIntechOpen, London, UK; 2017. https://www.inte chopen.com/chapters/54213

[3] Colberg SR, Sigal RJ, Yardley JE, Riddell MC, Dunstan DW, Dempsey PC, et al. Physical activity/exercise and diabetes: A position statement of the American Diabetes Association. Diabetes Care. 2016;**39**(11):2065-2079. DOI: 10.2337/dc16-1728

[4] Macera CA, Hootman JM, Sniezek JE. Major public health benefits of physical activity. Arthritis and Rheumatism. 2003;**49**(1):122-128. DOI: 10.1002/art.10907

[5] Musumeci G. Effects of exercise on physical limitations and fatigue in rheumatic diseases. World Journal of Orthopedics. 2015;**6**(10):762-769. DOI: 10.5312/wjo. v6.i10.762

[6] National Ataxia Foundation [Internet]. 2023. Available from: https://www.ataxia.org/change-to-nfl-concussion-protocols-brings-awareness-to-ataxia/

[7] Kramer A. An overview of the beneficial effects of exercise on health and performance. Advances in Experimental Medicine and Biology. 2020;**1228**:3-22. DOI: 10.1007/978-981-15-1792-1_1

[8] Smith PJ, Blumenthal JA, Hoffman BM, Cooper H, Strauman TA, Welsh-Bohmer K, et al. Aerobic exercise and neurocognitive performance: A meta-analytic review of randomized controlled trials. Psychosomatic Medicine. 2010;**72**(3):239-252. DOI: 10.1097/PSY.0b013e3181d14633

[9] Hamer M, Chida Y. Physical activity, and risk of neurodegenerative disease: A systematic review of prospective evidence. Psychological Medicine. 2009;**39**(1):3-11. DOI: 10.1017/S0033291708003681

[10] Hillman CH, Erickson KI, Kramer AF. Be smart, exercise your heart: Exercise effects on brain and cognition. Nature Reviews. Neuroscience. 2008;**9**(1):58-65. DOI: 10.1038/nrn2298

[11] Loprinzi PD. The role of astrocytes on the effects of exercise on episodic memory function. Physiology International. 2019;**106**(1):21-28. DOI: 10.1556/2060.106.2019.04

[12] Psychologicalscience.org [Internet]. 2023. Available from: https://www.psychologicalscience.org/uncategorized/myth-brain-training-will-make-you-smarter.html

[13] Maugeri G, D'Agata V, Magrì B, Roggio F, Castorina A, Ravalli S, et al. Neuroprotective effects of physical activity via the adaptation of astrocytes. Cell. 2021;**10**(6):1542. DOI: 10.3390/cells10061542

[14] Fabel K, Fabel K, Tam B, Kaufer D, Baiker A, Simmons N, et al. VEGF is necessary for exercise-induced adult hippocampal neurogenesis. The European Journal of Neuroscience. 2003;**18**(10):2803-2812. DOI: 10.1111/j.1460-9568.2003.03041. x

[15] Colcombe SJ, Erickson KI, Scalf PE, Kim JS, Prakash R, McAuley E, et al.

Aerobic exercise training increases brain volume in aging humans. The Journals of Gerontology. Series A, Biological Sciences and Medical Sciences. 2006;**61**(11):1166-1170. DOI: 10.1093/gerona/61.11.1166

[16] Erickson KI, Voss MW, Prakash RS, Basak C, Szabo A, Chaddock L, et al. Exercise training increases size of hippocampus and improves memory. Proceedings of the National Academy of Sciences of the United States of America. 2011;**108**(7):3017-3022. DOI: 10.1073/pnas.1015950108

[17] Reid G, Bouffard M, MacDonald C. Creating evidence-based research in adapted physical activity. Adapted Physical Activity Quarterly. 2012;**29**(2):115-131. DOI: 10.1123/apaq.29.2.115

[18] Lanza G, Casabona JA, Bellomo M, Cantone M, Fisicaro F, Bella R, et al. Update on intensive motor training in spinocerebellar ataxia: Time to move a step forward? The Journal of International Medical Research. 2020;**48**(2):1-15. DOI: 10.1177/0300060519854626

[19] Mandolesi L, Polverino A, Montuori S, Foti F, Ferraioli G, Sorrentino P, et al. Effects of physical exercise on cognitive functioning and wellbeing: Biological and psychological benefits. Frontiers in Psychology. 2018;**9**:509. DOI: 10.3389/fpsyg.2018.00509

[20] Song YG, Ryu YU, Im SJ, Lee YS, Park JH. Effects of dance-based movement therapy on balance, gait, and psychological functions in severe cerebellar ataxia: A case study. Physiotherapy Theory and Practice. 2019;**35**(8):756-763. DOI: 10.1080/09593985.2018.1457119

[21] Winser SJ, Pang M, Tsang WWN, Whitney SL. Tai chi for dynamic balance training among individuals with cerebellar ataxia: An assessor-blinded randomized-controlled trial. Journal of Complementary and Integrative Medicine. 2022;**28**(2):146-157. DOI: 10.1089/jicm.2021.0222

[22] Duret C, Breuckmann P, Louchart M, Kyereme F, Pepin M, Koeppel T. Adapted physical activity in community-dwelling adults with neurological disorders: Design and outcomes of a fitness-center based program. Disability and Rehabilitation. 2022;**44**(4):536-541. DOI: 10.1080/09638288.2020.1771439

[23] Rodríguez-Díaz JC, Velázquez-Pérez L, Rodríguez Labrada R, Aguilera Rodríguez R, Laffita Pérez D, Canales Ochoa N, et al. Neurorehabilitation therapy in spinocerebellar ataxia type 2: A 24-week, rater-blinded, randomized, controlled trial. Movement Disorders. 2018;**33**(9):1481-1487. DOI: 10.1002/mds.27437

[24] Sawant P, Gokhale P. Functional approach in spinocerebellar ataxia-occupational therapy perspective. Indian Journal of Physiotherapy & Occupational Therapy. 2015;**9**:222-227

[25] Salcı Y, Fil A, Keklicek H, Çetin B, Armutlu K, Dolgun A, et al. Validity, and reliability of the international cooperative ataxia rating scale (ICARS) and the scale for the assessment and rating of ataxia (SARA) in multiple sclerosis patients with ataxia. Multiple Sclerosis and Related Disorders. 2017;**18**:135-140. DOI: 10.1016/j.msard.2017.09.032

[26] Cernak K, Stevens V, Price R, Shumway-Cook A. Locomotor training using body-weight support on a treadmill in conjunction with ongoing physical therapy in a child with severe cerebellar ataxia. Physical Therapy. 2008;**88**(1):88-97. DOI: 10.2522/ptj.20070134

[27] Honório S, Batista M, Serrano J, Petrica J, Mesquita H, Ribeiro J, et al. Programa de ejercicios de intervención

para personas con ataxia motora. Retos; 2020;**38**:602-605. DOI: 10.47197/retos.v38i38.77614. Available from: https://recyt.fecyt.es/index.php/retos/article/view/77614/48907

[28] Weyer A, Abele M, Schmitz-Hübsch T, Schoch B, Frings M, Timmann D, et al. Reliability, and validity of the scale for the assessment and rating of ataxia: A study in 64 ataxia patients. Movement Disorders. 2007;**22**(11):1633-1637. DOI: 10.1002/mds.21544

[29] Freund JE, Stetts DM. Use of trunk stabilization and locomotor training in an adult with cerebellar ataxia: A single system design. Physiotherapy Theory and Practice. 2010;**26**(7):447-458. DOI: 10.3109/09593980903532234

[30] Ilg W, Synofzik M, Brötz D, Burkard S, Giese MA, Schöls L. Intensive coordinative training improves motor performance in degenerative cerebellar disease. Neurology. 2009;**73**(22):1823-1830. DOI: 10.1212/WNL.0b013e3181c33adf

[31] Kim BR, Lim JH, Lee SA, Park S, Koh SE, Lee IS, et al. Usefulness of the scale for the assessment and rating of ataxia (SARA) in ataxic stroke patients. Annals of Rehabilitation Medicine. 2011;**35**(6):772-780. DOI: 10.5535/arm.2011.35.6.772

[32] Pérez-Avila I, Fernández-Vieitez JA, Martínez-Góngora E, Ochoa-Mastrapa R, Velázquez-Manresa MG. Efectos de un programa de ejercicios físicos sobre variables neurológicas cuantitativas en pacientes con ataxia espinocerebelosa tipo 2 en estadio leve [Effects of a physical training program on quantitative neurological indices in mild stage type 2 spinocerebelar ataxia patients]. Revista de Neurologia. 2004;**39**(10):907-910 Spanish

[33] Milne SC, Corben LA, Georgiou-Karistianis N, Delatycki MB, Yiu EM. Rehabilitation for individuals with genetic degenerative ataxia: A systematic review. Neurorehabilitation and Neural Repair. 2017;**31**(7):609-622. DOI: 10.1177/1545968317712469

[34] Miyai I, Ito M, Hattori N, Mihara M, Hatakenaka M, Yagura H, et al. Cerebellar ataxia rehabilitation trial in degenerative cerebellar diseases. Neurorehabilitation and Neural Repair. 2012;**26**(5):515-522. DOI: 10.1177/1545968311425918

[35] Garcia V, José F, Barbado D, Moya MC. Trunk stabilization exercises for healthy individuals. Revista Brasileira de Cineantropometria e Desempenho Humano. Brazil: SciELO. 2014;**16**:200-211. Available from: https://www.scielo.br/j/rbcdh/a/CNY7jGZ4CC6hFfX9pvn4spy/?lang=en#

[36] Kitago T, Krakauer JW. Motor learning principles for neurorehabilitation. Handbook of Clinical Neurology. 2013;**110**:93-103. DOI: 10.1016/B978-0-444-52901-5.00008-3

[37] Widener GL, Conley N, Whiteford S, Gee J, Harrell A, Gibson-Horn C, et al. Changes in standing stability with balance-based torso-weighting with cerebellar ataxia: A pilot study. Physiotherapy Research International. 2020;**25**(1):e1814. DOI: 10.1002/pri.1814

[38] Cohen H, Blatchly CA, Gombash LL. A study of the clinical test of sensory interaction and balance. Physical Therapy. 1993;**73**(6):346-354. DOI: 10.1093/ptj/73.6.346

[39] Podsiadlo D, Richardson S. The timed "up & go": A test of basic functional mobility for frail elderly persons. Journal of the American Geriatrics Society. 1991;**39**(2):142-148. DOI: 10.1111/j.1532-5415.1991.tb01616.x

[40] Fitts PM. The information capacity of the human motor system in

controlling the amplitude of movement. 1954. Journal of Experimental Psychology. 1992;**121**(3):262-269. DOI: 10.1037//0096-3445.121.3.262

[41] Ilg W, Schatton C, Schicks J, Giese MA, Schöls L, Synofzik M. Video game-based coordinative training improves ataxia in children with degenerative ataxia. Neurology. 2012;**79**(20):2056-2060. DOI: 10.1212/WNL.0b013e3182749e67

[42] Schatton C, Synofzik M, Fleszar Z, Giese MA, Schöls L, Ilg W. Individualized exergame training improves postural control in advanced degenerative spinocerebellar ataxia: A rater-blinded, intra-individually controlled trial. Parkinsonism & Related Disorders. 2017;**39**:80-84. DOI: 10.1016/j.parkreldis.2017.03.016

[43] Levac D, Espy D, Fox E, Pradhan S, Deutsch JE. "Kinect-ing" with clinicians: A knowledge translation resource to support decision making about video game use in rehabilitation. Physical Therapy. 2015;**95**(3):426-440. DOI: 10.2522/ptj.20130618

[44] Synofzik M, Ilg W. Motor training in degenerative spinocerebellar disease: Ataxia-specific improvements by intensive physiotherapy and exergames. BioMed Research International. 2014;**2014**(583507):1-11. DOI: 10.1155/2014/583507

[45] Ziegle R. Adaptive Physical Activity for Students with Cerebral Palsy [Internet]. 2023. Available from: https://www.pelinks4u.org/articles/stopka/oct07_a.htm

[46] Sherrill C. Adapted Physical Activity, Recreation, and Sport: Crossdisciplinary and Lifespan. 6th ed. Boston: McGraw-Hill; 2004

[47] Fitnesslabco.com [Internet]. 2023. Available from: https://fitnesslabco.com/physical-therapy-clinic/balance-gait-disorders/

[48] World Health Organization (WHO). World Report on Disability. Geneva: World Health Organization; 2016

[49] Ellapen TJ, Hammill HV, Swanepoel M, Strydom GL. The health benefits and constraints of exercise therapy for wheelchair users: A clinical commentary. African Journal of Disability. 2017;**6**:337. DOI: 10.4102/ajod.v6i0.337

[50] Macpherson C, Bartsch B, King M, Kuo S-H, Quinn L. Engage-ataxia: Preliminary results after 1 year from a physical activity coaching intervention in individuals diagnosed with ataxia. In: Proceedings of the International Congress for Ataxia Research 2022, Dallas, USA. Takeda (www.taceda.com); 2022. p. 100. Available from: https://www.ataxiacongress.org/ICAR-2022-AbstractBooklet-PostConferenceVersion.pdf

[51] Tipton CM. The history of "exercise is medicine" in ancient civilizations. Advances in Physiology Education. 2014;**38**(2):109-117. DOI: 10.1152/advan.00136.2013

[52] Janssen I, LeBlanc AG. Systematic review of the health benefits of physical activity and fitness in school-aged children and youth. International Journal of Behavioral Nutrition and Physical Activity. 2010;**7**:40. DOI: 10.1186/1479-5868-7-40

[53] Mahindru A, Patil P, Agrawal V. Role of physical activity on mental health and well-being: A review. Cureus. 2023;**15**(1):e33475. DOI: 10.7759/cureus.33475

Chapter 6

Nutritional Care and Intervention in Spinocerebellar Ataxia

Donnette A. Wright

Abstract

This chapter examines the link between nutritional health outcomes in clients diagnosed with spinocerebellar ataxia as well as generalized quality of life and well-being that is achieved as a result of nutritional intervention and concordant nutritional status. Spinocerebellar ataxia is a familial disorder typified by degenerative changes to the neurological system including the brain, and spinal cord, impacting mobility and volitional actions. Due declining neural activity, the management of health and wellness in the affected individuals is central to mitigating the functional decline and morbidity. The linkage between dietary intake and nutritional support is a significant element of the health care interventions necessary to provide optimal health outcomes in clients diagnosed with spinocerebellar ataxia. Accordingly, an analysis of factors that impact dietary intake, and nutritional profile is pivotal in regulating disease progression, remission and management. The isochronous relationship between nutritional support and spinocerebellar ataxic progression and the concordant impact of disease progression on nutritional outcome is a critical subject for review. Lastly, summative standardized models are essential to guiding the health care strategy for managing the wellbeing of individuals with spinocerebellar ataxia.

Keywords: micronutrients, vitamins, minerals, neurological, nutrition care

1. Introduction

The global prevalence of spinocerebellar ataxia is 1 to 5 per 100,000 but higher in Asian populations while lower in European countries [1]. Ataxia is the loss of neural control over muscular tone and function affecting gait, coordination, eye movement, and speech; swallowing and other voluntary activities are also affected. Spinocerebellar ataxia (SCA) is a large and complex group of hereditary (genetic, familial), progressive, neurodegenerative, and heterogeneous disease that mainly affects the cerebellum. SCA is a subgroup of inherited cerebellar ataxia and is a rare disease. Currently, in excess of 40 distinctive genetic SCAs have been identified. The genetic contributions and impact of SCA is very complex to understand but is critical to diagnosing and classifying the disease which determine treatment approaches [1, 2]. SCA presents clinically with several symptoms related to the neuromuscular systems and is characterized by cerebellar gait and limb ataxia (with dysmetria, dysdiadochokinesia, intention tremor, dysarthria, and nystagmus), which may be present together with extracerebellar signs, such as ophthalmoplegia, pyramidal signs, movement disorders (including parkinsonism, dystonia, myoclonus, and chorea), dementia, epilepsy, visual disorders (including pigmentary retinopathy), and peripheral neuropathy. These symptoms contribute to significant physiological impact which influences Disability Adjusted Life Years (DALY). One DALY is the equivalent of one healthy life-year lost and contributes to the global disease burden [3, 4]. Individuals diagnosed with SCA may present clinically with self care deficits and experience increased nutrient requirements coupled with limitations in dietary intake. The progressive nature of the disease makes it critical for early nutritional intervention and management to correct, resolve and limit the negative health and nutrition outcomes associated with the disease. Consequently, health care practitioners must collaborate to create the best therapeutic outcome for the client diagnosed with SCA.

2. Overview of nutrition and neurological health

Nutrition is a key determinant of overall physical wellness and as a consequence specific neurological function and wellness. Nutrition has been identified as a strong modifier of healthy aging, body composition and physical function [5–7]. Through dietary intake, people acquire the related nutrients, substrates, and components necessary to maintain health and carry out life sustaining functions and reactions. To illustrate, a meal consisting of chicken provides protein to an individual who consumes it. Following digestion, deamination, transamination, and the Krebs cycle, proteins are catabolized either to energy in the form of adenosine triphosphate (ATP) or may enter the amino acid pool which produces substrates for physiological processes such as coagulation, immunity, muscle accretion or enzymatic support [8]. When nutritional adequacy is achieved through balanced dietary intake physiological homeostasis is attained and wellness equilibrium is established. Where dietary intake is discordant with requirements and nutritional needs remain unsatisfied, individuals may experience metabolic stress, catabolic changes and physiological impairments. This physiological wellness is a primary underpinning concept of overall wellness and is important for establishing optimum neurological status.

Furthermore, normal neurological status and functioning is a state that occurs when genetic, biological and physiological conditions are optimal. While genetic and biological conditions are largely non modifiable conditions; nutrition is an important regulatory on the physiological contributions to optimal neurological status. Importantly optimal neurological status requires a constant supply of some chemical substrates, known as neurotransmitters, which are essential to the typical signaling in the brain. Glutamate, glycine, γ-Aminobutyric acid (GABA) and acetylcholine are the key neurotransmitters in degenerative neurological disorders that are influenced by dietary intake. Spinocereballar ataxia (SCA) has been described as a heterogenous autosomal degenerative disease with multiple subtypes affecting both sensory and motor function with significant progressive decline which affects self care and independent functioning. The evidence suggests a clear genetic anomaly impacting the development of the condition. Some studies use metabolomics to identify associated biomarkers that are linked to the development of the disease. Metabolomics is a recent powerful scientific strategy used to identify and measure potential biomarkers, especially metabolites and small molecular weight molecules, in neurodegenerative diseases capable of determining alterations in brain function which can be affected by metabolite composition of biological fluids such as the serum, plasma, and cerebrospinal fluid. Amino acids including but not limited to Valine, Leucine, and Tyrosine have been linked to the development, diagnosis and sequencing of spinocerebellar ataxia [9]. Other evidence supports this finding but expands the report to include challenges with glutamine and calcium regulation as contributing metabolites to SCA development [10].

In some sub types of spinocerebellar ataxia, the evidence suggests that the ability to recover normal function reduces as the client ages and the disease develops. Therefore, recent studies recommend early therapeutic intervention for a better chance of having a positive neurological impact [11]. Molecular studies support these recommendations insomuch as they demonstrate that dietary amino acid intake produces substantial effects on health and disease by modulating metabolism. Recent studies have shown that newer dietary patterns, such as the ketogenic diet and the Paleo diet, have recorded clinical benefits on metabolic health, neural function, and longevity [12]. While the literature is expansive concerning the recommendations for carbohydrates and fats in health and wellness, protein requirements are usually given as a single nutrient recommendation rather than disaggregated by monomeric stratification. The current data proposes that amino acids, the building block of proteins, are unique in their functions and biological requirements are variable. Amino acids such as serine, glycine, asparagine, histidine, and methionine mediate health and disease including cancer and neurological disorders through defined molecular mechanisms [12, 13]. Some of these amino acids, histidine and methionine, are essential which means the human body lacks the biological capacity to make them and they must therefore be supplied by the diet. Others, though non essential and able to be made de novo, require sufficient substrates for development. This creates a unique conundrum for clients diagnosed with SCA because as the physiological need for amino acids rises, physical factors such as coordination and dependency limit their intake which may result in true or functional deficiency.

Consistent with these findings are the therapeutic recommendations which suggest that increased availability of these amino acids is beneficial to neurological health. Targeted pharmacological and therapeutic approaches have been consistently used to increase the availability of these amino acids in translation and gene expression, especially in neurological disorders, such as through induced pluripotent stem cell but not much has been done to explore and create consensus concerning the nutritional contributions of these amino acids in neuropharmacotherapy. The evidence suggests that foods such as eggs, cheeses, pineapples, nuts and seeds and salmon have been shown to significantly improve mental health outcomes [14]. These foods are high in tryptophan (an essential amino acid) that is critical to neurological activity. Similarly, dairy products including milk, cheese and dark chocolate, as well as eggs, beef, chicken, salmon, trout and legumes have been identified to be rich in histidine, methionine, leucine and other essential amino acids as well as the non essential serine that are linked to neurological health [15, 16]. Serine has been isolated as an important amino acid that modifies the health outcomes in neurological conditions affecting both sensory and motor activities [17].

Notably, dietary intake and interventions directly affects physiological health and mental wellness through its general supply of substrates of homeostasis. Specifically, diet supplies neurotransmitters necessary for the signaling of nerves. A concerted effort, of the multidisciplinary health care team, needs to be employed to ensure dietary adequacy for normal neurological functioning and to assist in recovery where sensory and motor neurological disorders exist.

2.1 Nutrient metabolism and brain health

Although the brain only accounts for two percent of the body's weight, it utilizes a quarter of the ingested energy of the human's body. It primarily utilizes glucose as the source of energy and so prefers carbohydrate as the main macronutrient source. It relies on aerobic respiration and oxidative processes for energy production and cellular activity [18]. An important part of neurons is the phospholipid coating that supports quick transmission of nerve impulses. Unlike organs such as muscles, liver and kidney, the brain has very limited energy stores and relies on a constant dietary supply of macro and micronutrients to meet dietary needs. The brain utilizes one fifth of the total blood glucose for daily functioning and only stores small amounts of glycogen in astrocytes. Carbohydrate promotes good mental health through its positive impact on dopamine levels, serotonin levels and its impact on cortisol release [18, 19]. Complex carbohydrates with lower glycaemic index and sustained energy provision in the blood are better suited to controlled energy supply to the brain.

Similarly fatty acids, phospholipids and polyunsaturated fatty acids such as linoleic acid and linolenic acid have been found to improve synaptic functions and cell signaling [18, 20]. Moreover, amino acids, the protein monomers, have been found to have both naturally positive and negative neuronal impact. Recommended intake of amino acids at physiological concentrations produce nitric acid, taurine and glutathione which promote good mental health but in excess amino acids produce metabolites that are neurotoxic including ammonia and homocysteine [18, 21].

Several studies have linked the B vitamin group to positive mental health outcomes and status. Thiamine, Riboflavin, Niacin, Pantothenic acid, Folate and Cyanocobalamin have all been positively linked to good mental health [18, 22]. These water-soluble vitamins influence and promote energy release as well as macronutrient metabolism, RNA and DNA formation and cellular signaling. Moreover, deficiencies in some of these vitamins have been linked to higher risks of mental illnesses including B9 (Folate) and B12 (Cyanocobalamin). Though energy balance is essential to neuronal homeostasis, current evidence suggests that dysfunctional energy metabolism as well as metabolic impairment may increase the risk of mental illness. The changes in the brain function, cell signaling, nerve conduction and brain activity alters energy utilization and requirements in mental illness [19]. Some evidence also points to risks of metabolic syndrome, impaired glucose tolerance and diabetes as conditions that can arise from muscle relaxant therapy as a part of the pharmacotherapy in spinocerebellar ataxia [23].

2.2 Nutritional requirements and brain health

Current evidence points to higher levels of prooxidant activity, reactive oxygen species and a concordant increased use of antioxidant in some subtypes of SCA. Consistent with this finding is the increased risk of being susceptible to oxidative stress and oxidative cellular damage [24, 25]. Clients with SCA7 exhibit oxidative damage to lipids (high levels of lipid hydroperoxides and malondialdehyde) and proteins (elevated levels of advanced oxidation protein products and protein carbonyls). Furthermore, SCA7 clients showed enhanced activity of various anti-oxidant enzymes (glutathione reductase, glutathione peroxidase, and paraoxonase) as well as increased total anti-oxidant capacity, which suggest that activation of the antioxidant defense system might occur to counteract oxidant damage. Furthermore, clients with degenerative neurological conditions have relatively higher requirements for antioxidants. These molecules are thought to be protective, especially in the neuronal spaces. It has been primarily linked to improved outcomes. Nutrients that are classified as antioxidants include zinc, selenium, ascorbic acid, retinol, and tocopherols. Fruits, vegetables, and fish provide concentrated sources of these nutrients. Additionally, polyunsaturated fatty acids have been strongly linked and examined in mitigating and treating mental illness. At recommended levels essential unsaturated fatty acids including linoleic and linolenic fatty acids support cell signaling, synaptic function and nerve impulse propagation. In degenerative disorders the evidence suggests that the demand for antioxidants is higher, the pathways are upregulated as well as the production of prooxidant species with relatively worsened clinical outcomes [24–26]. Consequently, consumption of fatty acids at the level of the recommended dietary allowances and fatty acid supplementation have been found to be beneficial in reducing the risks associated with mood disorders and have also been linked to improved recovery from these illnesses.

Some trace elements including zinc, copper and iron and manganese, have been associated with Neurological disorders. Some evidence also describes the link between zinc and neurological and the inverse relationship between zinc supplementation and the resolution of these symptoms [27–29]. Zinc has been associated with brain function and development and is also a potent antioxidant which combats the actions of prooxidants, superoxides and reactive oxygen species which negatively impact degenerative neurological disorders.

Individuals who experience SCA, have increased needs for nutrients including major minerals, trace elements, and antioxidants as their body utilizes these substrates at a faster rate in view of the increased brain activity. Consumption of high biological value sources, at the Recommended Dietary Allowances and supplementation have been strongly associated with lower illness incidence and better recovery.

2.3 Drug nutrient interaction and spinocerebellar ataxia

The health outcomes of SCA worsens as the disease develops with progressively worse motor and sensory activities with time. In addition to gene therapy as means of reducing and reversing the physical outcomes, clients diagnosed with degenerative neurological disorders are often treated with Riluzole, Antiglutaminergic Medication such as Amantadine, Nicotine Receptor Agonists such as Varenicline and Serotonergic Therapy among other pharmacological options [30, 31]. Collectively these medications may cause reduced appetite, vomiting, diarrhea, weight loss and anorexia and sore throat. While these symptomatic medication targets the improvement in the quality of life of clients affected by SCA, caution must be exercised with their use so that nutrition decline is not potentiated. Appetite loss and Anorexia may reduce the likelihood of clients meeting the recommended dietary allowances (RDA) and the acceptable macronutrient distribution ranges (AMDR) of key macronutrients carbohydrates, proteins and fats and important micronutrients such as zinc, copper, iron and manganese that have been linked to the physiological outcomes of the disease. Diarrhea and vomiting which are other significant side effects of these therapies may contribute to subclinical and clinical deficiencies as plasma levels decline with loss. Therefore, a collaborative holistic multi-team approach is necessary to treat SCA including the dietitian, pharmacist and the medical doctor.

2.4 Altered physical activity and energy metabolism in clients with degenerative disorders

There is a direct proportional relationship between energy requirements and physical activity. More energy is required in individuals who engage in physical activity whether voluntary or involuntary. Clients with neurological conditions, by virtue of the impact on the musculoskeletal system, may either be more or less active and directly have varying energy needs. Clients diagnosed with SCA may experience neurological impact resulting in hyperactivity characterized by involuntary movements. Individuals who are diagnosed with these conditions may experience tremors, muscle spasms and other movement disorders as symptoms of the condition. Moreover, the psychopharmacotherapy used in the treatment of spinocerebellar ataxia has negative side effects including tardive dyskinesia, restlessness and aggression. Alternatively, some clients exhibit reduction in motor activity and dysarthria, limited voluntary activity while on the same medications [11, 32]. These symptoms are at dipoles and require different nutritional therapeutic interventions to meet the physiological needs of the affected clients. In clients with reduced physical activity such as those who experience slow, sluggish movement, energy intake needs to be reduced to prevent obesity and positive energy balance while in clients who experience increased physical engagement as a consequence of increased involuntary activity, increased energy intake through the global increase of all macronutrients is the ideal nutritional therapy suited to these clients. Macronutrients are energy producing nutrients and include protein, carbohydrates and fats that are provided in the diet mainly from eating starches, animal and plant based foods and fruits. Due to the supportive role that micronutrients, especially water soluble B vitamins, play in macronutrient metabolism their requirements are also increased in accordance with energy requirements. These micronutrients serve as cofactors and coenzymes in energy metabolism so that energy can be increase from consuming the calorie containing foods [33]. Alternatively, another physiological feature of SCA, that results in reduced dietary intake is reduced swallowing capacity and coordination. This limits the client's ability to prepare food and feed themselves as well as to earn for the provision of meals. Additionally, dietary intake may be negatively affected by features of dependence and reliance on caregivers [11, 32]. Dietary modification such as textures; mechanically soft or pureed; are ideal for swallowing difficulties while nutrient dense economical meals, such as stewed legumes or low costs subprimal or retail animal, are recommended in financial resource restrictions.

Clients experiencing degenerative neurological disorders utilize higher or lower values of energy either due to the pathophysiology of the condition or the therapeutic cost of managing the condition. A personalized treatment approach is necessary dependent on the pole of the energy utilization spectrum that the client is on; higher energy intake is required in more metabolically active individuals and energy/calorie restrictions in individuals who consume or require less energy.

3. Final remarks and conclusion

Neurological degenerative disorders affect a relatively small segment of the global population but accounts for extensive disability in the affected cohort. The management of degenerative disorders has primarily surrounded pharmacotherapy, neurostimulation and gene therapy with little focus on nutritional therapy. Recent evidence suggests that this is likely due to the fact that the field of nutritional neurological research is relatively new [34]. Nevertheless, both classic and contemporary evidence points to a strong link between nutritional intake, status, and neurological health outcomes. Consequently, the management of degenerative neurological disorders should be comprehensive and include a multi-team approach. The team of health care workers who are essential to the nutritional wellbeing of clients with neurological disorders include the phlebotomist, physician, nurse, home care assistant and the dietitian. These team members must collaborate to assess, diagnose, prescribe, treat and support the nutritional needs of the ill client towards impacting his overall clinical outcome. The treatment plan is geared at client centered approach that matches nutritional interventions to the pathophysiological changes of the client with neurological disorders.

The main nutritional recommendations for the support and management of neurological disorders includes but is not limited to:

Multiteam collaborative support including a nutritionist and/or dietician to assess nutritional needs and status and create nutrition plans and interventions targeted and personalized to each client to support their recovery or prevent the occurrence. This approach ideally may reduce the course, progress, and outcome of the disease inasmuch as nutrition is employed as a therapeutic strategy. It includes the assessment of the clinical progress of the client, energy needs based on weight, physical activity and diseased state and matches the physiological needs of the client to the ideal nutrition care strategy for optimization of health. The nutrition prescriptions usually match both need for energy (from macronutrients) and the need for micronutrients.

The current evidence suggests worsening neurological decline in clients with SCA where energy and micronutrient intake may be below physiological level which negatively impacts health outcomes. This progressive decline affects dietary intake as well as nutrient requirements. A strategy to improve client overall health results is to offer healthy small packaged foods frequently especially to those exhibiting dependency and reduced appetite in order to limit dietary impact. Foods including dark chocolate, and cheeses have been found to be associated with improved neurological outcomes and meet the needs of clients who require more accessible options. Dark chocolate, in particular, has been found to improve antioxidant levels and is thought to positively affect prooxidant activities in these disorders [35].

For clients with specialized nutritional needs such as those with swallowing difficulties and increased needs for micronutrients, nutrition therapy is critical for recovery and improvement. One element of nutrition therapy is meal planning. Nutritional meal planning is an essential tool that can be utilized to support neurological health and recovery. Meal planning is a structured activity that involves forecasting and preparing nutritionally adequate meals designed to meet the dietary needs of clients. In the first instance, the principle and technique can be taught to the client by an expert and for sustained outcomes adopted and practiced by the affected clients.

The technique allows for energy balance, variety and moderation among other positive outcomes which are beneficial to mental health.

Routine biochemical assessments are essential to health maintenance and management of neurological disorders. Interventions, to be most beneficial, must be grounded in the evidence and client specific data. Biochemical tests may provide information concerning micronutrient status, deficiency or toxicities which are crucial for designing strategies to promote neuronal health and wellness and are likely risk factors in SCA with increased needs, utilization in the face of reduced intake. Some biochemical tests that may be beneficial in the assessment of SCA clients include Complete Blood Counts, Urea and Electrolyte analysis and Nutrition Panel as well as screens for other micronutrients. Results of biochemical analyses are critical for guiding the use of supplements.

Most of the plans to promote neurological health in SCA client addresses balance and increased intake but the comprehensive nutritional guide must also address targeted dietary restrictions such as energy restrictions in the face of inactivity or reduced physical activity.

Pharmacological side effects must be monitored and treated collaboratively to prevent a decline in nutritional status and the related biochemical impact in these diseases.

Finally, the group of clients affected by SCA forms a unique population of health care clients with physiological needs impacting biochemistry and functionality. These expand to present unique nutritional impact affecting status which is direct predictor of health outcomes. The management of the client with SCA must be multifaceted and incorporate nutrition as an essential therapeutic prong. The comprehensive targeted individualized nutritional support including client centered assessment, prescription, adjustment and evaluation, is the best strategy for the nutritional management of degenerative neurological disorders including SCA where the focus is on both micronutrient and macronutrient intake.

Author details

Donnette A. Wright
The University of the West Indies, Kingston, Jamaica

*Address all correspondence to: donnette.wright02@uwimona.edu.jm

References

[1] Bhandari J, Thada PK, Samanta D. Spinocerebellar ataxia. In: Stat Pearls [Internet]. Tampa, Florida, United States: StatPearls Publishing; 2022

[2] Teive HA, Munhoz RP, Arruda WO, Lopes-Cendes I, Raskin S, Werneck LC, et al. Spinocerebellar ataxias: Genotype-phenotype correlations in 104 Brazilian families. Clinics. 2012;**67**:443-449

[3] Chin JH, Vora N. The global burden of neurologic diseases. Neurology. 2014;**83**(4):349-351

[4] Murray CJ, Vos T, Lozano R, Naghavi M, Flaxman AD, Michaud C, et al. Disability-adjusted life years (DALYs) for 291 diseases and injuries in 21 regions, 1990-2010: A systematic analysis for the global burden of disease study 2010. The Lancet. 2012;**380**(9859):2197-2223

[5] Bales CW, Starr KNP, Miller M. Physical function and body composition as nutritional outcomes: Assessment approaches. Innovation in Aging. 2019;**3**(Suppl 1):S392

[6] Wright DA, Hewitt-Thompson KPG. Impact of Nutrition in Spinocerebellar Ataxia. IntechOpen: In Spinocerebellar Ataxia; 2021

[7] Starr KNP, Young K, McDonald SR, Loyack N, Lagoo-Deenadayalan SS, Heflin MT, et al. Nutrition assessment in high-risk patients: NRS-2002, PG-SGA, and NFPE in older adults preparing for elective surgery. Innovation in Aging. 2019;**3**(Supplement_1):S392

[8] Gupta A. Metabolism of proteins and amino acids. In: Comprehensive Biochemistry for Dentistry. Singapore: Springer; 2019. pp. 377-393. DOI: 10.1007/978-981-13-1035-5_13

[9] Nambo-Venegas R, Valdez-Vargas C, Cisneros B, Palacios-González B, Vela-Amieva M, Ibarra-González I, et al. Altered plasma acylcarnitines and amino acids profile in spinocerebellar ataxia type 7. Biomolecules. 2020;**10**(3):390

[10] Di Gregorio E, Borroni B, Giorgio E, Lacerenza D, Ferrero M, Buono NL, et al. ELOVL5 mutations cause spinocerebellar ataxia 38. The American Journal of Human Genetics. 2014;**95**(2):209-217

[11] Orr HT. Cell biology of spinocerebellar ataxia. Journal of Cell Biology. 2012;**197**(2):167-177

[12] Dai Z, Zheng W, Locasale JW. Amino acid variability, tradeoffs and optimality in human diet. Nature Communications. 2022;**13**(1):6683

[13] Piper MD, Soultoukis GA, Blanc E, Mesaros A, Herbert SL, Juricic P, et al. Matching dietary amino acid balance to the in silico-translated exome optimizes growth and reproduction without cost to lifespan. Cell Metabolism. 2017;**25**(3):610-621

[14] Sliwinska S, Jeziorek M. The role of nutrition in Alzheimer's disease. Roczniki Państwowego Zakładu Higieny. 2021;**72**(1):29-39

[15] Górska-Warsewicz H, Laskowski W, Kulykovets O, Kudlińska-Chylak A, Czeczotko M, Rejman K. Food products as sources of protein and amino acids—The case of Poland. Nutrients. 2018;**10**(12):1977

[16] Nurdiani R, Prihanto AA, Firdaus M. Seafood as source of protein-based functional foods. Encyclopedia of Marine Biotechnology. 2020;**133**:2987-2997

[17] Ye L, Sun Y, Jiang Z, Wang G. L-serine, an endogenous amino acid, is a potential neuroprotective agent for neurological disease and injury. Frontiers in Molecular Neuroscience. 2021;**14**:726665

[18] Raju MSVK. Medical nutrition in mental health and disorders. Indian Journal of Psychiatry. 2017;**59**(2):143

[19] Zuccoli GS, Saia-Cereda VM, Nascimento JM, Martins-de-Souza D. The energy metabolism dysfunction in psychiatric disorders postmortem brains: Focus on proteomic evidence. Frontiers in Neuroscience. 2017;**11**:493

[20] Bazinet RP, Layé S. Polyunsaturated fatty acids and their metabolites in brain function and disease. Nature Reviews Neuroscience. 2014;**15**(12):771-785

[21] Oswald MC, Garnham N, Sweeney ST, Landgraf M. Regulation of neuronal development and function by ROS. FEBS Letters. 2018;**592**(5):679-691

[22] Young LM, Pipingas A, White DJ, Gauci S, Scholey A. A systematic review and meta-analysis of B vitamin supplementation on depressive symptoms, anxiety, and stress: Effects on healthy and 'at-risk 'individuals. Nutrients. 2019;**11**(9):2232

[23] Bao YK, Ganesan VC, Jiang W, Lin L, Brown NR, Steigerwalt KE, et al. Muscle relaxant induced pancreatitis leading to hyperosmolar hyperglycemic state. Oxford Medical Case Reports. 2019;**2019**(3):omz 012

[24] de Assis AM, Saute JAM, Longoni A, Haas CB, Torrez VR, Brochier AW, et al. Peripheral oxidative stress biomarkers in spinocerebellar ataxia type 3/Machado–Joseph disease. Frontiers in Neurology. 2017;**8**:485

[25] Torres-Ramos Y, Montoya-Estrada A, Cisneros B, Tercero-Pérez K, León-Reyes G, Leyva-García N, et al. Oxidative stress in spinocerebellar ataxia type 7 is associated with disease severity. The Cerebellum. 2018;**17**:601-609

[26] Cornelius N, Wardman JH, Hargreaves IP, Neergheen V, Bie AS, Tümer Z, et al. Evidence of oxidative stress and mitochondrial dysfunction in spinocerebellar ataxia type 2 (SCA2) patient fibroblasts: Effect of coenzyme Q10 supplementation on these parameters. Mitochondrion. 2017;**34**:103-114

[27] Ferreira CR, Gahl WA. Disorders of metal metabolism. Translational science of rare diseases. 2017;**2**(3-4):101-139

[28] Squadrone S, Brizio P, Mancini C, Abete MC, Brusco A. Altered homeostasis of trace elements in the blood of SCA2 patients. Journal of Trace Elements in Medicine and Biology. 2018;**47**:111-114

[29] Tarnacka B, Jopowicz A, Maślińska M. Copper, iron, and manganese toxicity in neuropsychiatric conditions. International Journal of Molecular Sciences. 2021;**22**(15):7820

[30] Perlman SL. Update on the treatment of ataxia: Medication and emerging therapies. Neurotherapeutics. 2020;**17**(4):1660-1664

[31] Sarva H, Shanker VL. Treatment options in degenerative cerebellar ataxia: A systematic review. Movement disorders clinical practice. 2014;**1**(4):291-298

[32] Egorova PA, Bezprozvanny IB. Molecular mechanisms and therapeutics for spinocerebellar ataxia type 2. Neurotherapeutics. 2019;**16**(4):1050-1073

[33] Huskisson E, Maggini S, Ruf M. The role of vitamins and minerals in energy metabolism and well-being. Journal of International Medical Research. 2007;**35**(3):277-289

[34] Aucoin M, LaChance L, Cooley K, Kidd S. Diet and psychosis: A scoping review. Neuropsychobiology. 2020;**79**(1-2):20-42

[35] Tsang C, Hodgson L, Bussu A, Farhat G, Al-Dujaili E. Effect of polyphenol-rich dark chocolate on salivary cortisol and mood in adults. Antioxidants. 2019;**8**(6):149